Praise for *Matchless Organization*

"The story of the Confederate Army Medical Department has finally risen, phoenix-like, from the ashes of the great Richmond fire of April 2, 1865, which consumed the enterprise's voluminous and historically rich records. *Matchless Organization* is a tour de force recounting the organization, function, and fate of the Confederate medical service. Had other branches of the Confederate war machine worked as well as the medical department, the conflict's outcome might have been different."
　　　　—**Bill J. Gurley,** coauthor of *I Acted from Principle:*
The Civil War Diary of William McPheeters,
Confederate Surgeon in the Trans–Mississippi

"Well researched and well written, Hasegawa's book provides a scholarly account of the Confederacy's medical department under the leadership of Surgeon General Samuel Preston Moore. Organized thematically, it offers an insider's view into the department's operations and the versatility of its management. It is both innovative and thought-provoking."
　　　　—**John S. Haller Jr.,** author of *Battlefield Medicine: A History of the*
Military Ambulance from the Napoleonic Wars through World War I

"Hasegawa's overview of how the Confederate medical system developed and functioned (or not) over the course of the Civil War is concise, clear, and as complete as available sources allow. This is information that anyone who studies, or even encounters, Confederate medicine in any way will want to have at their fingertips.
　　　　—**Glenna R. Schroeder-Lein,** author of *Confederate Hospitals*
on the Move: Samuel H. Stout and the Army of Tennessee

ENGAGING
the
CIVIL WAR

Chris Mackowski and Brian Matthew Jordan, Series Editors

A Public-History Initiative of Emerging Civil War
and Southern Illinois University Press

MATCHLESS ORGANIZATION

THE CONFEDERATE ARMY MEDICAL DEPARTMENT

Guy R. Hasegawa

Foreword by F. Terry Hambrecht

Southern Illinois University Press
Carbondale

Southern Illinois University Press
www.siupress.com

24 23 22 21   4 3 2 1

Cover illustration: the pavilion-style Chimborazo Hospital, built on a plateau
    just east of the Richmond city limits (cropped). *Library of Congress
    (reprod. no. LC-DIG-ppmsca-33629)*.

Library of Congress Cataloging-in-Publication Data
Names: Hasegawa, Guy R., author. | Hambrecht, F. Terry, writer of
    foreword.
Title: Matchless organization : the Confederate Army Medical Department
    / Guy R. Hasegawa ; foreword by F. Terry Hambrecht.
Other titles: Engaging the Civil War.
Description: Carbondale : Southern Illinois University Press, [2021]
    | Series: Engaging the Civil War | Includes bibliographical references
    and index.
Identifiers: LCCN 2020038325 (print) | LCCN 2020038326 (ebook)
    | ISBN 9780809338290 (paperback) | ISBN 9780809338306 (ebook)
Subjects: LCSH: Moore, Samuel Preston, 1813–1889. | Confederate States of
    America. Army. Medical Department—History. | Confederate States
    of America. Surgeon-General's Office—History. | Surgeons general
    (Military personnel)—Confederate States of America—History.
Classification: LCC E546.7 .H37 2021 (print) | LCC E546.7 (ebook)
    | DDC 973.7/75—dc23
LC record available at https://lccn.loc.gov/2020038325
LC ebook record available at https://lccn.loc.gov/2020038326

Contents

Gallery beginning on page 95

Foreword

F. Terry Hambrecht, MD
Senior Technical Advisor to the National
Museum of Civil War Medicine

In 1911 former Confederate surgeon Deering John Roberts observed, "As the records of the Confederate hospitals were burned in the surgeon-general's office at the fall of Richmond, it is difficult at this date to write of their work." Dr. Guy Hasegawa faced the same challenge in writing *Matchless Organization*, but unlike Roberts, he could not draw on his own memories of the war or interview former Confederate medical personnel for their recollections. He has relied instead on primary-source materials, some of which were collected for his previous scholarly publications on Civil War medicine. *Matchless Organization*, like Hasegawa's other works, is based on extensive original research over many years. That prolonged experience has helped Hasegawa interpret his findings in the proper context.

Matchless Organization has a number of attributes that make it stand out in the field of Confederate medical literature, placing it on the level of H. H. Cunningham's classic *Doctors in Gray* while avoiding significant redundancy with that work. *Matchless Organization* contains a wealth of new information ferreted out by painstaking exploration of previously unrecognized or underused archival sources. Other authors have only superficially explored some of the more traditional sources, but Hasegawa has added important details that they missed. Principal among the unpublished materials he has used are those kept by the National Archives and Records Administration, Washington, DC, such as the correspondence of the Confederate surgeon general, secretary of war, and adjutant and inspector general. Hasegawa also draws on fascinating published sources that describe individuals and aspects of the Confederate Medical Department. These include the recollections of diarist Mary Chesnut, staff officer Gilbert Moxley Sorrel, and War Department clerk John B. Jones. Appendixes A and B provide capsule biographies of key players, including not only the personnel in the Surgeon General's Office but also individuals who interacted with and exerted authority over that office. Among the latter were

President Jefferson Davis, Adjutant and Inspector General Samuel Cooper, and the various Confederate secretaries of war.

The reader learns how Confederate officials sometimes bypassed the chain of command and interjected their strong personalities to obtain their goals or to deny those of others. One cannot help but conclude that the Confederate Medical Department was efficient and well organized but could have achieved more of its mission with additional help from the officials with authority over it. Also important were the department's interactions with the Confederate Congress, which at times tried to be helpful but was too often overridden by President Davis. Particularly fascinating is the account of how Confederate surgeon general Samuel Preston Moore and his senior staff, most of whom had served in the US Army Medical Department, had to educate the volunteer physicians who received commissions in the new Confederate medical service. Those formerly civilian physicians did not appreciate the importance of following military regulations regarding hygiene in camps and hospitals as a means of preventing disease. *Matchless Organization* clearly shows how the Confederate Medical Department achieved positive outcomes through applying the known principles of public-health reform, sanitation, and vaccination.

Although Surgeon General Moore had superb organizational ability and an overall understanding of the necessities of an efficient medical department, he was not without flaws. These were frequently pointed out as criticisms by persons who had to associate with him. Nonetheless, when the war was over, the general conclusion was that Moore had been an excellent choice for the position.

Future researchers in Civil War medicine will find the bibliography of *Matchless Organization* to be a major asset. More than 250 sources are listed. Yet beyond the titles themselves is the information gleaned from those references and woven into the narrative. I was not previously aware of some of the sources despite being a student of Civil War medicine and surgery for over fifty years. Hasegawa also points out questions that his research has not answered, which will serve as guideposts for future scholars on the subject.

Readers might yearn for more personal information about Samuel Preston Moore, his family, and his life in the US Army before the American Civil War. Moore was not an outgoing man and did not share this type of information in his very limited papers and presentations. He did not write an autobiography and evidently kept no journal or diary, which obviously would have been very helpful.

I highly recommend *Matchless Organization* for those interested in learning more about the American Civil War and the Confederate Medical Department in particular.

Preface

When former Confederate surgeon Francis Peyre Porcher addressed a gathering of wartime colleagues in 1899, he paid tribute to the late Samuel Preston Moore, a fellow South Carolinian who had served for most of the Civil War as the Confederate army's surgeon general. In citing Moore's creation of "the matchless organization of the medical department of the Confederate army," Porcher echoed a view expressed consistently by other former Southern medical officers—the Confederate Medical Department was extraordinarily well arranged and owed its efficiency to Moore.

Given the many disadvantages faced by the South during the Civil War, it is remarkable that the Confederate army was able to survive as long as it did against an opponent that had the upper hand in manpower and materiel. One factor having a profound effect on any army is its health, so the Medical Department of the Confederate army merits study not only for its efficiency but also because what it did was so important.

For the general reader, learning about Confederate military medicine should start with H. H. Cunningham's *Doctors in Gray*, first published in 1958 and still the standard introduction to the topic. Cunningham presented a wide view of Confederate medicine, from actions taken in the Southern capital to maladies suffered by common soldiers in the field. His decision to provide a panorama prevented him from delving deeply into any particular aspect of Confederate military medicine, so while he described decisions made in the Surgeon General's Office (SGO), he stopped short of giving readers an inside view of the operation.

My aim in *Matchless Organization* is to explore the Medical Department as an organization and the SGO as its administrative core. By describing the setting in which the department operated, I hope to provide enough context to allow readers to understand the otherwise confusing actions taken by it or imposed upon it by other government entities. *Matchless Organization* offers information from sources not used by other historians (for example, records of the secretary of war and adjutant and inspector general, letters from the SGO to members of Congress, and amnesty records) and documents its references fully, which *Doctors in Gray*—because of unfortunate publication decisions—does not. Even the most avid of Civil War enthusiasts may find some unfamiliar facts in *Matchless Organization* and be enabled to research them further. This book also centers on Richmond, not only because that city housed the SGO but also because management decisions concerning the Medical Department had the greatest influence there. Compliance with orders emanating from the capital tended to diminish with distance from Richmond. In addition, forming conclusions about activities west of the Mississippi River presents challenges because of the scarcity of relevant records about that region of the Confederacy.

I have not attempted in *Matchless Organization* to cover Southern naval medicine or to explore in detail every aspect of army medicine. Although there have been studies of Confederate general hospitals—for example, the excellent *Confederate Hospitals on the Move*, by Glenna Schroeder-Lein—enough original records survive to support more research into that topic and others, such as the army's medical-purveying operations. *Matchless Organization* covers the middle ground between very specific studies and the wide-ranging *Doctors in Gray*.

Samuel Preston Moore, who took command of the Medical Department in July 1861, plays the most prominent role in this book. Although several articles have been written about him, a full-length biography has not appeared, probably because no researcher has found enough information about him to fill a book. *Matchless Organization* is not a biography but describes Moore's actions as surgeon general and examines the factors that steered his decisions.

Moore's job required that he be a master of multitasking. Many things were happening simultaneously and influencing each other, and he had to eschew a tunnel-vision approach in favor of one that considered all related factors. One could truly appreciate his position only by being there and living it in real time. Since that is impossible, I have organized topics thematically and, within those themes, presented events in roughly chronological order. This approach, which comes with the caveat that Moore's considerations were complex and interconnected, necessitates some redundancy and cross-referencing, which I hope readers will find more helpful than distracting. Other personalities also played vital and sometimes multiple roles. Appendix A is offered to assist readers in keeping these individuals and their positions straight.

Many of the records kept at the SGO were scattered at the end of the war or destroyed by the fire that consumed much of Richmond in early April 1865. Yet records survive from Richmond facilities that were outside of the fire zone and from medical personnel, hospitals, and offices dispersed throughout the

South. Relatively few truly explanatory documents—for instance, reports by Moore to the president or the secretary of war—are available to help elucidate the thinking behind various actions. Many documents examined for this book are letters, and even in the rare cases in which complete exchanges are available, proper interpretation requires an appreciation of the relevant context. *Matchless Organization* contains some educated guesses, but I have based them on the best information available and identified speculation as such.

I am grateful to the many individuals who assisted with this project. Among the most helpful, I must single out F. Terry Hambrecht, MD, who has been a mentor from the start of my Civil War research more than twenty years ago and encouraged me to write this book. Terry has, with Jodi Koste of Virginia Commonwealth University, been compiling an unpublished register of physicians who served the Confederacy in a medical capacity; information from that source, freely shared by Terry, has been highly valuable. He also provided his painstakingly created transcriptions, also unpublished, of wartime letter books containing communications of Confederate surgeon J. J. Chisolm and other medical officers. Terry, an expert on Confederate medicine, acted as a sounding board as I developed this book, and he reviewed its manuscript. He was the obvious choice to write the foreword.

Important assistance also came from Jonathan O'Neal, MD, a long-time student of Confederate medicine, who shared his knowledge of the South's general hospitals, provided documents and photographs from his collection, and commented on the book manuscript. Debra Chisolm Ruehlman generously shared copies of correspondence involving her ancestor Dr. Chisolm and allowed the use of his wartime photograph. Ray Nichols graciously provided his transcriptions of National Archives records of Confederate medical purveyors; his generosity spared me from untold hours of tedium. Numerous librarians and archivists, particularly at the National Archives, patiently aided me in retrieving records. Susan Hoffius of the Waring Historical Library, Medical University of South Carolina, and Rosemary Spellman of the Library Services Center, Sheridan Libraries, Johns Hopkins University, merit special thanks for their assistance. Sylvia Frank Rodrigue, executive editor for Southern Illinois University Press, once again helped me navigate the publication process and gave expert advice on how to improve the manuscript.

Finally, I could not have written this book without the encouragement and patience of my wife, Betsy, and our sons, David and Stephen, who have supported my historical endeavors from the start.

Matchless Organization

ENGAGING
—the—
CIVIL WAR

For additional content that will let you engage this material further, scan the QR code on this page. It will take you to exclusive online material and related blog posts at www.emergingcivilwar.com.

A QR scanner is readily available for download through the app store on your digital device. Or go to www.siupress.com/matchlessorganizationlinks for links to the digital content.

Introduction

As the newly declared Confederate States of America began to take shape in early 1861, its leaders had no way to anticipate the optimal organization of the various bureaus of the War Department. Unknown at the time were whether armed conflict would actually occur and, if so, for how long it would last and to what scale it would be fought. How effective would the Union naval blockade be, and would European powers recognize and aid the Confederacy? Without such recognition, would the Southern states have the resources to survive on their own? How would the doctrine of states' rights affect the ability of the Confederate military to wage war as a unified force?

Despite lacking answers to these and other vital questions, Southern leaders could look to a convenient model of government—that of the United States. Thus, the first law adopted by the Confederate States called for continuation of all US laws that were not inconsistent with the Confederate Constitution. The War Department took the same approach by initially modifying the 1857 US Army regulations and, to the extent possible, filling its positions with men who had recently served in the US military.[1]

The new secretary of war, Leroy Pope Walker, had confidently asserted during the secession debate that there would be no serious armed conflict and that he would be able to wipe up any spilled blood with his pocket handkerchief. The Provisional Confederate Congress seemed to agree when it initially allowed the appointment of army surgeons and assistant surgeons in numbers that would be woefully inadequate should major fighting occur. Newly appointed medical officers were sent to various posts even before an overall department leader, in the form of a surgeon general, was identified and appointed. On assuming his post, the army's first acting surgeon general did not know exactly where his officers had been assigned and had to ask Walker, who lacked meaningful military or medical expertise, how much medicine to buy.[2]

How the Medical Department of the Confederate army operated is a story of improvisation and reaction to circumstances. Even those few medical officers who had recently served in the US Army had not seen military action conducted on the scale that the American Civil War would assume. The rest of the physicians—the vast majority—who would serve as medical officers had been civilian practitioners and entered upon their military duties knowing little about maintaining sanitation in camp, treating battlefield injuries surgically, managing the illnesses of an army, or completing the necessary forms and reports. In fact, the basic intellectual, physical, and moral fitness of those medical men had to be established. Sizable hospitals for military casualties were absent in the South before the war, as were the means of transporting large numbers of sick or wounded soldiers to medical facilities. The Southern states faced the unfamiliar circumstances of being primarily on the defensive and largely deprived of traditional sources of supply, the latter complicated by the lack of a robust industrial base and what would become a crippling inflation rate.

The Medical Department could not act in isolation and depended especially on cooperation from the Quartermaster and Subsistence Departments. It was subordinate to the president and secretary of war, and the influence—both enabling and interfering—of the Confederate Congress was a constant presence. In common with the other components of the Confederate military enterprise, the Medical Department suffered from worsening shortages of human and material resources. Given the imperfect means of communication, the diversity of circumstances throughout the South, and the ad hoc nature of how army organizations and procedures developed, it is no surprise that official decisions were sometimes unworkable, confusing, contradictory, or simply disregarded. Uniformity of effort among the various government entities in Richmond was difficult enough, but added to that was the wariness of individual states of any powerful central government and the desire of those states to exercise their will and maintain their identity.

To the extent that the Medical Department was allowed to control its operations, its efficiency depended on the quality of its organization and its management and on the adroitness with which it could adjust to a fluid environment. The department, which would eventually count thousands of men and women among its workforce, looked to the surgeon general to determine how to best meet the medical needs of an army of raw recruits spread over vast areas. That administrator, lacking previous experience in commanding a large group of subordinates, would direct a corps of medical officers, hospital stewards, and other caregivers whose civilian background left them initially unprepared to treat wartime injuries and illnesses and ignorant of military procedure and discipline. Clearly, the Confederate Medical Department had an enormous challenge ahead of itself. Its endeavor to optimize care and contribute to the war effort, described in the following pages, had its modest beginnings in the first capital of the Confederacy— Montgomery, Alabama.

1. ❖ Medical Department for a New Nation

The Medical Department of the Confederate army was established on February 26, 1861, to consist of one surgeon general with the rank of colonel, four surgeons with the rank of major, and six assistant surgeons with the rank of captain, all to be appointed by the president with congressional advice and consent. (Used generically, "surgeon" was a catchall term that encompassed all army medical officers, whether they performed surgical operations or not. But "surgeon" and "assistant surgeon" were also military grades that corresponded with ranks.) Those officers were part of the regular (permanent) army and, like their counterparts in the regular US Army, received an actual (rather than assimilated) rank; they would presumably remain in the service after the cessation of any hostilities. Additional assistant surgeons—as many as deemed necessary—were allowed at the same time, although whether they were to be in the regular army remains unclear. On April 25, about two weeks after the bombardment of Fort Sumter, Adjutant and Inspector General Samuel Cooper recommended adding six surgeons and fourteen assistant surgeons to the regular army. On May 16 President Davis approved a bill that expanded the total number of allowable regular-army positions in the Medical Department, other than the surgeon general, to ten surgeons and twenty assistant surgeons.[1]

Other legislation approved by Davis allowed the appointment of one surgeon and one assistant surgeon per regiment to help care for the large numbers of volunteer troops soon to swell the ranks of the army. Those supplemental positions were in the newly formed Provisional Army of the Confederate States (PACS), which would cease to exist after the anticipated conflict ended and the number of troops dropped to peacetime levels. Further legislation allowed the president to appoint as many medical officers in the PACS, who would receive the same pay and emoluments as their counterparts in the regular army, as were needed in hospitals. Because legislation mentioned no actual rank for them, assistant surgeons and surgeons in the PACS were considered to have the assimilated rank of captain and major, respectively. Not having actual rank had few practical ramifications, although it evidently wounded the self-esteem

4

of some of those who served. After the war, Edwin S. Gaillard, who had a dis-
tinguished record as a PACS surgeon, blamed Davis for the slight. "It was one
of the peculiarities of this great man," said Gaillard, "to deprive the medical
officers of the army of their actual rank." Medical officers in the PACS wore
the same uniform and insignia as their regular-army counterparts, although
the propriety of doing so was questioned by some Confederate senators. The
small number of regular-army slots meant that almost all Confederate medical
officers had an appointment in the PACS only.[2]

President Davis, having graduated from the US Military Academy and
served as US secretary of war, was well familiar with military matters and
practices. He believed that the chiefs of the various War Department bureaus,
of which the Medical Department was one, should have "special knowledge
of the duties to be performed," a prerequisite best met by "service creditably
rendered in the several departments of the United States Army before resigning from it." One army tradition—that of promoting officers or appointing
them to important posts on the basis of seniority—was, in fact, supported by
an act of the Provisional Confederate Congress. (The unicameral Provisional
Congress was replaced by the bicameral permanent Congress on February
18, 1862.) That act, passed on March 14, 1861, provided that all officers who
resigned from the US Army and received appointments in the regular service within six months would have their Confederate commissions bear the
identical date. That meant that the relative rank of such officers of the same
grade would be determined by how long they had held their rank in the US
Army. Thus, it seemed that the highest post in the Confederate Medical
Department, that of surgeon general, was destined for the highest-ranking
medical officer to resign from the US Army and be accepted into the regular
Confederate army by September 14. Beside the Medical Department, the
other original constituents of the army's general staff were the Adjutant and
Inspector General's Office (AIGO), the Quartermaster Department, and the
Subsistence (or Commissary) Department, with the head of each entitled to
the rank of colonel.[3]

On January 1, 1861, the US Army counted among its medical officers
a surgeon general, thirty surgeons, and eighty-three assistant surgeons. By
January 1, 1862, three full surgeons—Samuel Preston Moore, David Camden
DeLeon, and Thomas C. Madison—had resigned, and twenty-three assistant
surgeons had resigned or been dropped or dismissed from the US Army. Of
those twenty-six, twenty-three served as Confederate surgeons. They were
joined by at least two physicians—Francis Sorrel and Robert Southgate—who

had resigned their position as army medical officers some years before the Civil War. If there were no more such examples, then the grand total of former US Army surgeons to serve as Confederate surgeons was twenty-five.[4]

David Camden DeLeon: First Acting Surgeon General

Since President Davis was originally allowed to appoint four surgeons in the regular army, he first offered the positions in late March 1861 to the two men who had already resigned their commissions as full surgeons in the US Army—Moore, who declined, and DeLeon, who accepted—and then to former US Army assistant surgeons Edward W. Johns, William W. Anderson, and Elisha P. Langworthy.[5] Davis did not name a surgeon general with the March group of appointments but had an order issued on May 6 to have DeLeon—who had the longest service among the available medical officers—report to Montgomery, Alabama, the Confederacy's first capital, to assume the duties of acting surgeon general. When additional surgeon and assistant surgeon positions in the regular army became available later that month, Davis allotted them to the remaining former US Army surgeons. All of the assistant surgeons in the regular army received, at some point, concurrent appointments as full surgeons in the PACS, but the sequence of those appointments did not always parallel the officers' previous seniority in the US Army.[6]

DeLeon, a South Carolinian, entered the US Army in 1838 as an assistant surgeon. He served during the Second Seminole War, which ended in 1842, and earned the nickname "Fighting Doctor" during the Mexican War (1846–48) for twice leading troops after their commanding officers had been killed or wounded. During that conflict, he rode at the side of Major General Winfield Scott into Mexico City. DeLeon was promoted to surgeon in 1856 and was stationed for about seven years in New Mexico as a medical purveyor, an officer responsible for obtaining and distributing supplies.[7]

On February 19, 1861, DeLeon, then in Washington, DC, submitted his resignation and was reportedly summoned by General Scott, now the US Army's highest-ranking officer. According to DeLeon, Scott tried to dissuade Southern officers from resigning by promising them distant assignments that would preclude them from fighting in an impending civil war. DeLeon, given a few hours to choose between being arrested or accepting a posting to the northwestern frontier, quickly packed his trunk and left to serve the Confederacy. His first assignment as surgeon in the regular Confederate army was to direct the medical staff under Brigadier General Braxton Bragg at Pensacola.

When he received the call to report to Montgomery as acting surgeon general, he was in New Orleans serving as a medical director and medical purveyor. Once in the capital, he established an office in a "large and commodious fireproof building" rented to house the various departments of the Confederate government. The structure, located on the corner of Commerce and Bibb Streets and occupied, in part, by the Montgomery Insurance Company, was described by a British correspondent as "a large red brick building of unfaced masonry, which looks like a handsome first-class warehouse." DeLeon's brother called it "a great, red brick pile."[8]

DeLeon had made it known shortly after his resignation from the army that he wanted the position of surgeon general, and being named acting surgeon general was a step in the right direction. He had some reason to be optimistic. DeLeon had met Davis in 1860 (possibly earlier) and had friends in high places. During the interval between his appointment as acting surgeon general and the government's move to Richmond, which started at the end of May, he shared a Montgomery house with General Cooper (adjutant and inspector general and the highest-ranking officer in the army), Lieutenant Colonel Abraham Myers (acting quartermaster general), Lieutenant Colonel George Deas (an assistant adjutant general and inspector general), and others, including DeLeon's brother, Thomas. The house's piazza became the favorite place for "the better and brighter elements of the floating population" of Montgomery. DeLeon's title of acting surgeon general may have suggested that the only barrier to a permanent appointment was congressional approval. Alternatively, his appointment may have been considered pending until September 14, after which any surgeon who had been senior to him in the US Army could not have that seniority applied in the Confederate service. In any event, Samuel Preston Moore—who had outranked DeLeon and had earlier declined an appointment as surgeon in the regular Confederate army—wrote to the AIGO on May 4 about being appointed surgeon general. The details of that letter, received by the AIGO on May 13, or of any discussions about such an appointment are unknown. Also unknown is whether General Cooper, who surely knew about communications with Moore, mentioned them to his housemate.[9]

During DeLeon's brief tenure, Surgeon Edward W. Johns was assigned to temporary duty in the Surgeon General's Office (SGO), or the Medical Bureau, as it was sometimes called. After the move to Richmond on about June 1, Johns left the SGO to serve as Richmond's medical purveyor, while Surgeon Charles H. Smith and Assistant Surgeon Charles Brewer were assigned to the SGO; Johns, Smith, and Brewer all had appointments in the regular army. In Richmond, the War Department, including the SGO, first occupied the Custom House on Bank Street but moved about July 1 to the Virginia Mechanics Institute building on Ninth Street. A July 1861 Richmond directory indicated that the SGO staff included two clerks—listed as "S. G. Capers, M.D.," and "Wm. Duxberry"—and messenger Thomas Johnston. Capers was civilian physician Le Grande G. Capers Jr., who was said after the war to have been "one of the most useful coadjutors of the late Surgeon-General David Deleon in organizing the Medical Department of the Confederate Army" before becoming an assistant surgeon later in July. Duxberry may have been William C. Duxbury, a druggist from Montgomery who later became a Confederate artillery officer. The two men may also have staffed DeLeon's Montgomery office.[10]

Just after the SGO's move to Richmond, James M. Holloway of the Eighteenth Mississippi Regiment visited DeLeon with a paper signed by regimental officers recommending his appointment as surgeon in the Confederate service. Holloway described the encounter:

> I presumed he was the proper officer to take charge of my credentials. The old doctor was very kind and would have been pleased to serve me, but he had no authority to appoint; did not know to whom I should apply; had no list of surgeons already appointed; had thus far received no reports from the field, nor from the hospitals; in fact, was expecting daily the arrival of other medical officers of the old army who outranked him, and to one of whom he would have to turn over all he had, the nominal position of Surgeon General.

Holloway eventually received an appointment from the AIGO on June 11.[11]

Available records say little about DeLeon's overall performance as acting surgeon general. When he assumed that role, the Medical Department was unorganized, and confusion reigned. On May 1, just five days before assuming his duties, DeLeon was informed by the AIGO—probably in reference to regimental medical officers—that only assistant surgeons (no full surgeons) had so far been appointed. By July 1 DeLeon had urged, at least twice, the appointment of surgeons for regiments that were then being raised. On June 5 he informed the secretary of war that "most of the regiments now arriving [in Virginia] are totally unprovided with medical supplies; and from examination since my arrival here I am satisfied that those . . . in the field are for the most part in the same condition." At about the same time, DeLeon asked if he could select competent clerks for his office, such men being much needed. Nevertheless, according to DeLeon's brother, by mid-June 1861 the department had been "thoroughly reorganized and placed on really efficient footing," with hospitals and medical depots in Richmond "put in perfect order . . . under the personal supervision of the Surgeon-General."[12]

Notwithstanding that rosy assessment, a complaint arose about the acting surgeon general failing to supply troops in Virginia. In a possibly related action, DeLeon was relieved of his duties on July 12 and ordered to report to Norfolk, Virginia, to assume the role of medical director and medical purveyor for the Department of Norfolk. Temporary charge of the Medical Department would fall to Surgeon Charles H. Smith, who was, after DeLeon, the most senior of Confederate surgeons. DeLeon immediately asked President Davis to suspend the order until a court of inquiry could be ordered to investigate the aforementioned complaint. Davis deferred a decision only until he could learn more about the allegation. At the same time, DeLeon refused to turn over the SGO to Smith. Secretary of War Leroy P. Walker told DeLeon that nothing could be done until the surgeon showed "a disposition to recognize . . . [the War Department's] authority, and obey its lawful orders." DeLeon immediately softened his tone, told Walker he would obey, and presented an appeal: "It seems to me that the orders requiring me to serve under a junior must be a mistake. I know that you cannot intend to degrade an old officer. I throw myself on your view of justice and right." (At the time, *any* medical officer whom DeLeon might serve under would be his junior in terms of seniority.)[13]

Amid those exchanges, during which the First Battle of Manassas occurred (July 21, 1861), DeLeon continued his duties as acting surgeon general. He asked Walker, for example, how much quinine he should instruct a medical purveyor to purchase. The secretary, in his endorsement of the letter, instructed a subordinate to "address letter to 'Acting Surgeon Genl,'" which suggests a temporary suspension of the order relieving DeLeon from that office. DeLeon also signed himself as acting surgeon general when he responded to a July 20 request from Walker to estimate expenses for medical supplies. On July 24 he informed the AIGO that he was turning over the Medical Department to Smith but wished to defer his departure for Norfolk until he could settle some departmental accounts. That request granted and accounts settled, DeLeon reported a week later of his arrival for duty at Norfolk. No evidence has been found that a court of inquiry was convened.[14]

According to one report, a physician who had volunteered his services on the Manassas battlefield went to the SGO to report how poor the medical response had been in the battle's aftermath and to request supplies. There he met "two or three prim, scented dandies, who hardly treated him with respect." When the physician asked for the surgeon general, "he was told by these exquisites that they were 'all Surgeon Generals there.'" The accuracy of this account is unknown, but in the few days after Manassas, there might well have been confusion about who was really in charge. After all, DeLeon had been asked, more than a week after being relieved, to perform the duties of surgeon general, and Smith's expected role as temporary head of the SGO was probably anything but clear.[15]

The Department of Norfolk, of which DeLeon became the medical director, was absorbed into the Army of Northern Virginia in April 1862. Command of that army was assigned to General Robert E. Lee on June 1, 1862. DeLeon, who was recognized as senior medical officer, was named the army's medical director on June 3, taking the place of Surgeon Thomas Henry Williams, who would later serve in the SGO. In late June 1862, while on the battlefield during the Seven Days' Battles near Richmond, DeLeon was thrown from his horse and disabled. On June 27 Lee, after first offering the position to Surgeon Edward Warren, appointed Surgeon Lafayette Guild as acting medical director to replace the injured officer. Guild's appointment was later made official after consideration was also given to Surgeon Francis Sorrel to fill the spot. In a letter dated July 1862, DeLeon submitted his resignation from the army; it was accepted on August 1. How he spent the rest of the war is unclear. An 1872 obituary stated that the surgeon was "transferred to another department, and to various places during the war." Two accounts from the early twentieth century, one from a cousin, said that he served in the Trans-Mississippi Department, while an 1863 letter written by Confederate surgeon James Hunter Berrien in Texas referred to an invoice for medicines submitted by a Dr. DeLeon.[16]

The Arrival of Samuel Preston Moore

During the time that DeLeon was settling accounts in late July 1861, diarist Mary Chesnut observed that he was "always drunk." According to her, men hoping to assume his office included Robert Wilson Gibbes, a physician and naturalist in civilian life and now surgeon general of South Carolina, and Mobile surgeon Josiah Clark Nott. On July 26 Samuel Preston Moore checked in to the Spotswood Hotel in Richmond, and by July 28 it became general knowledge that he would be replacing Surgeon Smith, whose time in charge of the

SGO lasted about a week. The official order assigning Moore to that post was issued on July 30. What was behind Davis's decision to replace DeLeon with Moore is unclear. The president may simply have been honoring the seniority tradition by appointing Moore, whose commission as full surgeon in the US Army had preceded DeLeon's by seven years. Indeed, Dr. Sorrel, who served on Moore's staff in the SGO, said that Moore was "the ranking officer" at that time. DeLeon's obituary implies that, "under Mr. Davis's rule" (of seniority), it was only Moore's sudden availability that pushed DeLeon out as surgeon general. It may be relevant, too, that DeLeon's appointment as surgeon in the regular army was discussed and ultimately rejected by Congress; all other regular appointments of surgeons or assistant surgeons received congressional approval. In naming a surgeon general, it seems clear that Davis was unlikely to give serious consideration to men who had little or no military experience, such as Drs. Gibbes and Nott, regardless of their civilian accomplishments.[17]

Samuel Preston Moore was born in Charleston, South Carolina, in 1813; graduated from the Medical College of the State of South Carolina; and entered the US Army as an assistant surgeon in 1835. He served at a variety of military posts on the frontier, married in 1845, accepted a promotion to surgeon in 1849, and helped manage his late father-in-law's estate in Arkansas. During his service in the Mexican War, he impressed Davis, an army officer, with his skill as an organizer and disciplinarian. Moore's letters to his property agent in Arkansas reveal his disgust with politics and politicians and his disappointment with the remoteness of his army postings, aspects of the seniority system, the deceit of his superiors, and fellow officers who advanced themselves through the influence of powerful friends. Even if he were disposed to use such influence, said Moore, he did not know many important people who could help him. More than once he contemplated resigning from the army and taking up civilian medical practice in Arkansas. Among his antebellum responsibilities were serving on a medical examining board in Philadelphia with two future US Army surgeons general, Clement A. Finley and Charles H. Crane. In June 1860 Moore and his wife lost their eleven-year-old daughter to diphtheria. Although not a hot-blooded secessionist, the physician favored Southern independence and, after the 1860 election of Abraham Lincoln as US president, decided that he would soon resign from the army and move his family to Little Rock.[18]

Moore's final posting in the US Army was at New Orleans, where he was ordered on January 30, 1861. He arrived there before that date, for on the twenty-eighth, two days after Louisiana seceded from the Union, an official of the state militia demanded that the army surgeon surrender the medical department at New Orleans and its property. Moore complied, stating, "I have not the means of resisting this authority." The items yielded were eventually turned over to none other than future acting surgeon general DeLeon, who, as a newly appointed Confederate surgeon, had arrived from Pensacola to procure supplies. On February 12, writing from Magnolia, Mississippi, Moore submitted his resignation to US surgeon general Thomas Lawson. On the twentieth Henry L. Webb, who had commanded Moore during the Mexican War, wrote to President Davis to recommend his appointment as a Confederate surgeon.[19]

Moore recounted what happened after his resignation: "I went immediately after to Little Rock, Arkansas, to reside, and entered on the practice of my profession. I was offered the position of Surgeon in the C.S. Service in March 1861, which I did not accept." That offer was sent to the forty-seven-year-old on the twenty-sixth, with orders to report in person to the AIGO in Montgomery. It appears that, perhaps as a result of "the persistent appeals of his dearest friends, and from a high sense of duty," discussions took place by May that culminated in Moore's appointment as acting surgeon general in late July 1861. He was appointed surgeon general on November 7, which the Provisional Congress confirmed on December 13.[20]

The Surgeon General and His Bureau within the War Department

On paper the Medical Department was at the same level as the AIGO, the Quartermaster Department, and the Subsistence Department, with the heads of all four being of equal rank (colonel) and reporting to the secretary of war. But when Cooper was appointed adjutant and inspector general, he first was given the rank of brigadier general and then, on August 31, 1861, was promoted to full general, the first officer with that rank and making him the highest-ranking general in the Confederate army. Cooper, a confidant of Davis, was considered by the president to be the army's chief of staff and sometimes bypassed his nominal superior, the secretary of war, by dealing directly with Davis in making appointments and issuing orders. The Quartermaster Department was originally placed under the directorship of Lieutenant Colonel (later Colonel) Myers, who was replaced in 1863 by Brigadier General Alexander R. Lawton. The Subsistence Department was directed for most of the war by Colonel Lucius B. Northrop, whom President Davis promoted to brigadier general in November 1864; Northrop was replaced by Brigadier General Isaac M. St. John in February 1865. Thus, all of the departments constituting the army's original general staff, except the Medical Department, were led at one time by a full or brigadier general; Surgeon General Moore never attained a rank higher than colonel. According to historian Frank Vandiver, Moore "never seemed to be considered at the same level with the other service chiefs. . . . In the thinking of the other staff officers, he was a cut below them."[21]

Any hopes that Moore may have had for constancy in the chain of command were fleeting, for during his tenure in the SGO, which lasted throughout the war, the Confederacy had six different secretaries of war. Furthermore, President Davis considered himself a military expert and tended to take charge of tasks that might, under a different commander in chief, be handled by the secretary of war or the secretary's subordinates. Davis was also prone to applying the strict rule of law even when circumstances called for improvising or bending the rules. Thus, in trying to forward the aims of the Medical Department, Surgeon General Moore would have to deal with challenging personalities occupying a command hierarchy that may not have been entirely clear.

Within the Medical Department itself, the surgeon general's wishes could be carried out through the issuance of his own orders or circulars. Some actions, such as changes in personnel postings, were communicated through special or general orders issued by the AIGO in response to requests from the SGO. Actions that affected the Medical Department's relationship with other departments might require legislation or at least the approval of the secretary of war before they could be announced through the AIGO. Alteration of conditions established in legislation—such as the number, type, and rank of personnel assigned to the Medical Department—required additional legislation from the Confederate Congress and approval by the president. Although Congress generally seemed willing to assist the Medical Department, enactment of bills that would seemingly enhance the department's effectiveness was far from automatic.[22]

Attempts to elevate the responsibilities and status of medical officers began early. On December 17, 1861, Surgeon Charles Smith, a member of Moore's SGO staff, wrote directly to President Davis to clarify a previous discussion between the two. Smith expressed the desire of surgeons and assistant surgeons for authority to command noncommissioned officers and privates. Although medical officers were not then—or later during the war—allowed to exercise command outside of the Medical Department, Davis acknowledged that the need for such authority could arise and might warrant consideration. Perhaps Smith's comfort in suggesting legislation came, in part, from his observing the process during his prewar posting in the office of the US surgeon general in Washington, DC.[23]

A bill that reached Davis's desk (H.R. 29) in 1862 included provisions that Moore had previously suggested and that earlier pieces of legislation had failed to progress. It called for the rank of brigadier general in the PACS to be "conferred on the surgeon-general of the same"; for the appointment, also in the PACS, of two assistant surgeons general—one evidently intended to serve on either side of the Mississippi River—and one medical inspector general, all with the rank of colonel; and for up to twelve medical inspectors with the rank of lieutenant colonel. The bill called for the assignment of medical officers to other important positions.[24]

President Davis proclaimed his agreement with the aims of the act but vetoed it on October 13, 1862, because of obvious flaws. Among them was the fact that there was no such position as surgeon general in the PACS—Moore's appointment was in the regular army—so no officer existed on whom to confer the rank of brigadier general. In addition, the bill called for the *assignment* of a large number of medical officers without first allowing for enough men be given *appointments* as medical officers in the PACS.[25]

It is unclear where Davis stood on approving legislation that elevated the status of the Medical Department. Historian Wilfred Buck Yearns concluded that the president's preference "to let the [Medical] Department work out its own problems" discouraged Congress from taking action in that direction. In contrast, Robert G. Cleland and E. Merton Coulter separately noted that when Davis used his veto prerogative, it was when bills were unconstitutional, technically flawed, or clearly unwise. H. H. Cunningham concluded that H.R. 29, in particular, was poorly crafted and should have been vetoed. In any event, Moore would be disappointed if he hoped that raising the standing of the Medical Department would be accomplished easily through acts of Congress.[26]

Moore, whose years of army service must have accustomed him to coping with the resources at hand and circumstances as they presented themselves, could still manage the operations of this own department despite lacking the degree of support he desired. One indicator of that ability was the organization of his own office in Richmond.

2. ✸ The Surgeon General and His Office

As part of the War Department, the SGO was housed in the building of the Virginia Mechanics Institute—built in 1858—on Ninth Street between Main and Franklin Streets in Richmond, facing Bank Street and the southwest corner of Capitol Square, the grounds of the State Capitol. The "commodious" building, whose "style and execution [was] worthy of any cause or a place in any city," also contained the Navy Department and Patent Office. Within a few weeks of taking office, Moore complained that the single room he was allotted on the second floor was insufficient, requesting that two adjoining rooms be vacated by the Navy Department and attached to his outfit. Offices of the various War Department bureaus were to be open from 9 A.M. to 3 P.M. President Davis knew that bureau chiefs frequently left before three o'clock for dinner and directed Secretary of War Judah P. Benjamin to instruct the chiefs and their subordinates to observe official office hours.[1]

The SGO Staff

An unofficial government directory published in July 1861 showed Moore having an assistant surgeon general, two clerks, and a messenger but probably understated the size of the SGO staff, since Moore was entitled to at least fourteen clerks. Records suggest that SGO staff, including medical officers, grew to a maximum of about forty in early 1864; a detailed list at the end that year showed a total staff of thirty-five (see Appendix B). Among its members were civilian clerks and army personnel, primarily hospital stewards, detailed to work for the surgeon general. As the war progressed, women started to take the place of those men sent to serve in the field. Four women started working in the SGO in December 1863; that number increased to eleven in September 1864 and stayed at about that level until the end of the war.[2]

SGO holdovers from Moore's predecessor, DeLeon, included Surgeon Smith and Assistant Surgeon Brewer. Charles Henry Smith, a Virginian, had served in the US Army as an assistant surgeon since 1847. One of his last postings before resigning on April 25, 1861, was a short stint in the office of Surgeon General Thomas Lawson in Washington, DC. According to one of his colleagues in the Confederate SGO: "'Charley Smith' was surgeon and chief assistant. There was no such officer as 'Assistant Surgeon-General,' but he was always so considered and designated." Indeed, that title never existed officially, but it was applied to Smith in various publications throughout the war and in at least one official SGO communication in late 1864.[3]

Charles Brewer, native of Maryland, had served in the US Army as an assistant surgeon since 1856. He said shortly after the war that poor health and failure to secure a leave of absence prompted him to resign on April 21, 1861, and to seek health and employment as a private physician in Virginia. Unable to find a job, he accepted an appointment as assistant surgeon in the regular Confederate army, was promoted to surgeon in early 1862, and served almost exclusively in the SGO. While there he was termed the "assistant specially in charge of records of conscription, examining validity of exemptions, and general business of the office." When Richmond was evacuated in April 1865, Brewer was relieved from duty in the SGO and placed in charge of the eight thousand sick and wounded men left behind in the city's military hospitals, tasked with transferring their care to Federal authorities. Brewer's frail health accounted for him being the only medical officer on Surgeon General Moore's immediate staff to be designated unfit for field service. According to Assistant Adjutant General John Withers, Brewer and Moore assisted Surgeon Arthur E. Peticolas in amputating the arm of Surgeon Edwin S. Gaillard, a medical director wounded on May 31, 1862, at the Battle of Seven Pines. The operation occurred at Richmond's Spotswood Hotel, probably at the newly established hospital there.[4]

Moore arrived in Richmond only thirteen months after losing his daughter, and by the end of the war, Smith and Brewer would also be devastated by family deaths. In October 1862 Smith's five-year-old daughter died. Brewer's brother Isaac, a Confederate artillery officer, was killed in action in August 1862. In 1864 Brewer lost both parents, his brother Richard—a Confederate infantry officer also killed in action—and his two-year-old daughter. On May 12 Brewer was at the bedside of Major General James Ewell Brown Stuart when the cavalryman died of a wound sustained at the Battle of Yellow Tavern. Stuart's wife and Brewer's wife were sisters, and the mortally wounded general had been transported to the surgeon's residence in Richmond. Brewer's house was on the same block of West Grace Street as that of Surgeon General Moore.[5]

Joining Smith and Brewer in mid-August 1861 was Surgeon Francis Sorrel of Georgia. Sorrel had joined the US Army as an assistant surgeon in 1849, resigned in 1856, and moved to California to seek adventure. As a member of the California legislature, he was part of the minority voting for secession. Once the legislature adjourned in June 1861, Sorrel made his way back east to Richmond and received an appointment as surgeon in the regular army. He was the older brother of Gilbert Moxley Sorrel, perhaps best known as chief of staff for Lieutenant General James Longstreet. As a member of the SGO, Dr. Sorrel served as "assistant in charge of reports and records of sick and wounded, and inspector of hospitals in Richmond." He occupied a separate office on Bank Street near Ninth Street, a short walk from Moore's office in the Mechanics Institute building. There, with the assistance of Herman Baer and "a corps of disabled soldiers and clerks," Sorrel prepared "volumes of classified and tabulated gun-shot wounds and injuries, which were destroyed by the fire at the final evacuation."[6]

At least two additional medical officers are known to have joined the SGO staff. Thomas H. Williams of Maryland had served as an assistant surgeon in the US Army before submitting his resignation in May 1861. He was medical director of the Confederate Army of the Potomac and the Army of Northern Virginia before being displaced from the latter in June 1862 by former acting surgeon general DeLeon. The well-regarded Williams subsequently served as a hospital inspector and as temporary medical director for Major General Gustavus W. Smith's command before reporting for duty in January 1863 at the SGO, where he remained throughout the war. He was Moore's "assistant in charge of purveying business of the Medical Bureau."[7]

The last medical officer known to work in the SGO was Surgeon Herman Baer, who was born in Germany in 1830 and settled in Charleston, South Carolina, in 1847. Baer worked as a typesetter, tutor, and teacher and graduated in March 1861 from the Medical College of the State of South Carolina. He worked as a contract surgeon at a Richmond hospital before being appointed assistant surgeon, and later surgeon, in the PACS. By early 1864 he appears to have joined the SGO, where he collaborated with Sorrel in "tabulating and arranging statistics of reports of sick and wounded, certificates for retirement, and examining inspection reports."[8]

How Moore interacted with the other medical officers in the SGO is unclear. The surgeon general classified the services of all five as "absolutely indispensable," and he certainly would have transferred any of them whom he found inefficient or incompatible with his way of working. Gilbert Moxley

Sorrel described his brother Francis as Moore's "close confidential assistant" and noted that "the pair were forever rolling cigarettes."[9]

In November 1864 Moore and his five medical officers were assisted by eleven soldiers detailed for clerical duty and eight male and ten female civilian clerks. The women employed in the SGO included Elizabeth S. "Bettie" Saunders, bride-to-be of Lieutenant Colonel Walter H. Taylor, a member of General Robert E. Lee's personal staff. Most of the soldiers and male clerks were disabled or otherwise unfit for field service, as was typical for men assigned to government office work. Seven of the eleven soldiers were hospital stewards, noncommissioned officers who were often assigned as surgeons' assistants. Several of the men were members of the Third Regiment of Richmond's Local Defense Troops. One of them, Harry C. Morris, described having to drill every Wednesday afternoon, "the Department closing for that purpose." In late 1864 Morris's prolonged absence from the SGO while on duty with the troops near Chaffin's farm, Virginia, caused his office assignments to become "very much disordered," but Surgeon General Moore's plea to have Morris returned was denied.[10]

Richmond resident Sarah Ann Brock, perhaps having spoken with Bettie Saunders or her coworkers, claimed that Moore was held in high esteem by the clerks in his office. "Scrupulously exacting of them the strictest performance of duty," she wrote, "it was so well regulated as to make it a pleasure, while the slightest neglect of duty, we are told, was never permitted to pass unnoticed by him." Hospital Steward George W. Sites complained that clerking in the SGO was "the same thing every day, and you feel like a man in a tread-mill, or a horse turning a threshing machine." Referring to Hospital Steward Charles P. Bragg, an SGO clerk, Sites said, "I expect the poor fellow has learned what it is to *work* in the office of the Surgeon General, and if so, he has been benefited."[11]

Hard work in the SGO was surely needed to keep track of and manage the thousands of men and women who constituted the workforce of the Medical Department. During the decades after the war, estimates of the number of Confederate medical officers—or to be more precise, the number of positions filled by medical officers—arrived at a total of about 3,000. Those estimates probably undercounted positions in general hospitals and did not account for turnover. A modern register compiled by F. Terry Hambrecht and Jodi Koste suggests that about 7,400 men served as Confederate medical officers; many did not serve for the entire war. Although unknown, the number of hospital stewards was probably in the thousands. Numbers of other Medical

Department employees in early 1865 were reported as 1,083 men unable to perform field duty, 107 detailed conscripts, and 43 men detailed as contractors or artisans. Paul Van Riper and Harry Scheiber placed the department's peak employment of civilians at 8,250 persons, including 150 contract surgeons; 1,500 nurses, cooks, and stewards; 1,300 ward masters; 1,800 matrons; 1,500 laundresses; and 2,000 African American laborers. Their estimate for contract surgeons is well below that of Hambrecht and Koste (about 1,000).[12]

The Person of Samuel Preston Moore

An admiring 1863 article in the *Southern Illustrated News* described Surgeon General Moore, who had recently turned fifty, as a man "of medium height, scrupulously neat in his person and apparel . . . said by those who know him well to be genial in conversation, and of the very kindest disposition." In an apparent attempt to achieve a modicum of journalistic balance, the article added that the surgeon general possessed "official manners deemed by some abrupt." In fact, it was that abruptness that characterized Moore to most people who wrote about their wartime encounters with him.[13]

There were many such meetings between surgeons and Moore because all medical officers passing through or visiting Richmond, whether on duty or on leave, were required to report in person to the SGO. Surgeon John H. Claiborne described such a call on the surgeon general: "He took my card when I handed it to him, and without giving me any sign of recognition, threw it away." He then left him standing for a few minutes, reported Claiborne, before the surgeon general "lit a cigarette, which he made extemporaneously, and motioned for me to sit down." After a short interview, Moore sent him away to wait for orders, which were long in arriving. Assistant Surgeon Samuel C. Gholson reported a similar type of meeting, with Moore initially ignoring him and finally telling him to write his name in a book and return later for orders; he called Moore "surly, abrupt, and a martinet." Gholson's uncle, on hearing of the encounter, said that the surgeon general was equally unwelcoming with all callers, including Vice President Alexander Stephens and Secretary of War James Seddon, "but he was polite enough when he found that Mr. Stevens [*sic*] was his visitor." Even Surgeon Francis Peyre Porcher, whom Moore would grow to respect highly, reported that the surgeon general had treated him "under the appearance of great coldness" during their first meeting. After Porcher introduced himself, Moore looked up and told him nothing more than to return in the morning.[14]

Moore expected hard work not only from his office staff but also from other medical officers. "Leaves of absence must not be granted for trivial reasons," he told Surgeon William A. Carrington, medical director of Virginia's general hospitals. "It is not seen why a medical officer serving in hospital desires a leave of absence. The names of all supernumerary officers in hospitals of Richmond will be forwarded to this office for assignment." Surgeons not needed in hospitals, he noted, would be sent to the field. Medical officers in field were typically in short supply and unlikely to be underworked.[15]

One of Moore's approaches to undisciplined medical officers was to threaten them. In late September 1861 he issued a circular announcing that hospital surgeons not filing the proper reports would be reported to the president. The next month he stated that surgeons who were in charge of hospitals and failed to inform company commanders when their hospitalized soldiers were returned to duty would, "by direction of the Secretary of War, be reported to the President *for dismissal.*" Medical Director Thomas H. Williams believed that such measures were futile. "It is useless to report, or even threaten to report the Medical Officers of our Army for their seeming indifference to the Regulations," he wrote to Moore in November 1862, "as most of them occupy prominent social positions, and tender their resignations, as soon as they conceive their dignity invaded." Williams thought that more could be accomplished "by persuasion and by representing to them personally, the necessity that exists for prompt compliance with the requirements of the service, than by appealing to their fears." Moore, having neither the time nor inclination to apply such tactics in individual cases, issued a circular several weeks later instructing medical directors "to report to this office for the action of the Secretary of War, the names of all Medical Officers failing to render the Reports and Returns required by the Regulations, within five days after they become due."[16]

In another instance, Moore asked Secretary of War George W. Randolph to drop from the rolls "such medical officers who shall in the future in face of the enemy abandon their surgical instruments." He worried about the shortage of instruments, knew that many had already been lost by surgeons fleeing the battlefield, and thought "that the presence of medical officers on the field of battle without these instruments is as useless as that of soldiers unprovided with arms." Randolph directed the AIGO to order commanders to report the names of medical officers who lost their instruments or attempted to discharge their duties without them. That, at least, was a step short of summary discharge from the army.[17]

Moore's threats were not idle. When a board of surgeons granted furloughs of a length not allowed in regulations, he ordered those officers arrested and court-martialed. Before pressing charges, the AIGO sought and received an explanation—the details of which are unknown—from the president of the offending board. After reading the explanation, Moore agreed to withdraw the charges. In doing so, he revealed that he was willing to modify a previous judgment rather than stubbornly following through with it.[18]

After the war, Porcher explained that Moore's years of being "trained in the army, with all its ideas of discipline, its rigidity, and its formality," may have "deprived his manners . . . of that softness and suavity which are used in representative democracies and in all non-military communities." Within the SGO, he declared, Moore was an autocrat who seemed "cold and forbidding" and instilled fear into his subordinates. Nevertheless, Porcher did not consider him to be "cruel, arbitrary, or insensible to conviction." Even Surgeon Claiborne, who called the surgeon general "a man of great brusqueness of manner," acknowledged that Moore was "an able executive officer, and I believe an efficient and impartial one." Sarah Brock credited Moore's irreproachable record as surgeon general and characterized him as "polite and courteous, though so remarkably sententious that his manner was mistaken for unfeeling indifference." She maintained that he was best approached with "a simple statement of business" without "unnecessary preamble." Members of Richmond's city council thought of Moore as "a first rate man of business" but with "a very disagreeable way of showing it." Public opinion of his competence was generally high, but this was not a universal view. A North Carolina soldier who wrote periodically to a Fayetteville newspaper described the surgeon general as "a sour looking individual, some 50 yrs. old, a harsh, profane man, not possessing in my judgment qualifications and disposition requisite for that position."[19]

The surgeon general was not one to bow meekly to the opinions and actions of high-ranking officers. Adjutant and Inspector General Cooper claimed authority as the army's highest-ranking officer to make decisions for Moore (see chapter 3), and if the surgeon general took issue with Cooper's actions, he usually seemed to keep his concerns to himself. But, as described in later chapters, he did not hesitate to officially air his displeasure with General Lee's recommendation to close more general hospitals, with General Joseph E. Johnston's machinations to control general hospitals, or with General Bragg's attempt to remove men who had been detailed to a medical-purveying depot.

Moore was responsible for issues of huge complexity and importance, yet he could concern himself with seemingly trivial matters. When Surgeon James Brown McCaw, professor at the Medical College of Virginia (MCV) and director of Chimborazo Hospital, paid eighteen dollars for wood out of his hospital fund instead of obtaining it from the Quartermaster Department, Moore disallowed the transaction and cited the paragraph in army regulations that McCaw had violated. It was important that medical officers account properly for their expenses, but Moore had employees to check accounts and knew the hospital director to be highly efficient. In this instance he learned that McCaw had to skirt regulations because the quartermasters were so inefficient and ended up citing his predicament in a report to the secretary of war. Thus, although Moore could be quick to chastise officers for apparent neglect of regulations, he was willing to accept reasonable explanations. Much of the correspondence emanating from the SGO was probably dictated by one of Moore's subordinates, but the surgeon general personally signed most of it. That task, in itself, would have taken considerable time if he read the letters before signing. Moore even signed form letters notifying medical officers that they were delinquent in submitting reports.[20]

Former surgeon James M. Holloway described Moore as "thoroughly posted as to the duties of his position, and fully alive to the importance of thorough discipline in order to elevate the standard of the medical department and render it more effective." The surgeon general, he recalled, brought to his job "all the energies of a well-trained mind and inflexible will and untiring body" and was unsurpassed in "the quantity of mental and physical labor endured" during the war. According to Holloway:

No paper, letter, report, or order passed through his office without receiving his personal inspection and indorsement. He not only quickly grasped the purport of a paper, but, when written by a medical officer, he critically examined the diction, style, chirography and even the spelling. . . . The report of a surgeon that had been forwarded through my office was returned with the indorsement of the Surgeon General calling attention to misspelled words. At first this would seem to be pedagogical on the part of an officer at the head of so important a branch of the service, but not so when it is remembered that the Surgeon General . . . was determined that the effectiveness of his branch . . . would be demonstrated by close attention to detail.[21]

In one instance, Medical Purveyor George S. Blackie sent to the SGO, as required, a copy of a receipt for a few articles he had acquired from another purveyor. Moore returned the receipt with a note saying that, because the number of items was small, Blackie should have used "letter or foolscap paper" instead of expending a large, official preprinted form. In Moore's defense, paper was scarce and not to be wasted, but Blackie must have wondered whether he might just as easily have been chastised for failing to use a form.[22]

For all of his sternness, Moore could display a caring quality. When a hospitalized Union prisoner begged Secretary of War Randolph to be paroled and sent home so he would not contract a dangerous infection in his wound, the surgeon general personally accompanied Medical Inspector Sorrel to examine the patient. Chaplain William A. Crocker visited Moore to ask his help in compiling a list of hospitalized soldiers and their locations—this to aid patients' friends and family in finding their loved ones. The surgeon general deemed the project impractical but eventually gave Crocker permission to try, asked for progress reports, and offered any assistance within his power. The interaction left Crocker seeing the surgeon general as a "noble and kind-hearted old Southern gentleman." When a worried mother asked him to transfer her sick son to Chimborazo Hospital, Moore took the trouble to learn that the patient was stable and under proper care before sending a reassuring, yet characteristically formal, response. Moore also was not above acknowledging good work. When he learned of the commendable management of hospitals by Surgeon Dudley D. Saunders, he wrote, "Surgeon Saunders and the corps of medical officers will please accept the thanks of this office for the creditable manner in which they have performed their duty." Although Moore's gratitude was expressed with stiff formality, Saunders must have been pleased that his hard work had been noticed and officially recognized.[23]

That the surgeon general cared deeply about the welfare of Confederate soldiers is demonstrated by his continued efforts to improve the quality and organization of his department and thus the health of troops. While Moore's primary duty may have been to maximize the fighting strength of the army, he also showed concern for those who could no longer take up arms. In September 1862, for example, he suggested to Secretary of War Randolph the establishment of a facility for the "proper maintenance and protection" of disabled soldiers and officers, many of whom were without means or had a home in possession of the enemy. Moore believed that comfortable houses could be supplied at inconsiderable cost and that the venture could be operated as a "complete or semi-military organization" that would "secure to the invalids for the remainder of their lives, the consciousness of still being remembered by a grateful country." For convenience, he called the organization a "Military Asylum," but, as the term might be "unpleasant in its signification to so many of our people," proposed "Invalid Soldiers Home" or "Veterans Home" as an alternative. Shortly thereafter, the House of Representatives instructed its Committee on Military Affairs to investigate the expediency of Moore's proposal, but no legislation followed immediately.[24]

The idea arose again in late 1863, perhaps in response to a public entreaty from Reverend Charles K. Marshall, who was recognized for his efforts to assist sick or wounded soldiers. On December 28, 1863, Congressman Jeremiah W. Clapp of Mississippi introduced a bill that provided for a veteran soldiers' home. The next day Moore sent to Seddon, the current secretary of war, a copy of his previous communication to Randolph and asked him to forward it to Congress "to show the action taken by this Bureau on the subject, as well as to secure the attention of Congress in this matter." Marshall supported the bill and predicted that the "powerful influence" of Surgeon General Moore would help make it a success. Congress passed the measure in early February 1864, but President Davis vetoed it on the grounds that its proposed means for management and funding were unconstitutional.[25]

Moore also served as a director of the Association for the Relief of Maimed Soldiers (ARMS), a civilian group devoted to supplying artificial limbs to Confederate soldiers and sailors who had undergone amputation. Established in January 1864 at the urging of Reverend Marshall, ARMS also counted Surgeons McCaw and Charles Bell Gibson among its directors. Surgeon Carrington was the corresponding secretary of ARMS and essentially ran the organization, despite its having civilian officers headed by Marshall as president. Carrington, Moore, and McCaw were appointed as a committee to oversee all ARMS business other than matters relegated to a separate finance committee. Carrington used his army position to help obtain supplies for limb manufacturers with ARMS contracts and bent official rules—no doubt with the knowledge of Moore, who was usually a stickler for regulations—to make personnel assignments and transportation arrangements that would assist the association's contractors and help amputees obtain limbs.[26]

Even before his involvement with ARMS, Moore participated in another way to help provide artificial limbs. In November 1863 the War Department dispatched Surgeon John T. Darby to Europe to procure prostheses for various Confederate generals who had undergone amputation. Because high-quality artificial limbs could not be obtained in the South, he took castings of the generals' stumps to ensure that manufacturers would craft the prostheses to fit properly. Moore gave Darby various instructions or orders to supplement those imparted to him orally by the secretary of war.[27]

Moore and Politics

One trait mentioned with some consistency in accounts of Surgeon General Moore was his preference to avoid politics.[28] Holloway summarized why Moore's administration of the Medical Department drew condemnation:

> He was severely criticized oftentimes, and by officers in various branches of the service, and by members of Congress and other distinguished civilians, first, because he would not leave the duties of his office in the hands of subordinates and clerks and exercise his personal influence in having measures passed through Congress for the benefit of the Medical Department, and because, second, when visited by these distinguished gentlemen for the purpose of setting aside general orders to suit special cases the Surgeon General compelled them to take their turn in the line of visitors, and curtly refused special favors unless they appealed to his reason.[29]

The extent to which Moore tried to influence congressional action is undetermined. He did, at times, provide written information to legislators and encourage the writing and passage of bills that would help the Medical Department, apparently forming an early rapport with William Porcher Miles, chairman of the Committee on Military Affairs of the Provisional Congress and of the same House committee in the permanent Congress. After the war Moore characterized Congress as "appearing willing always to aid the [Medical D]epartment in its efforts towards a more perfect organization." Perhaps the major barrier to legislation that Moore favored took the form of vetoes by President Davis, which prompted him to conclude, "it seemed useless to make further efforts in this direction."[30]

The surgeon general also dealt with politicians who sought special consideration for their constituents. Congressman Franklin B. Sexton of Texas, for example, visited Moore in February 1863 about the commission of a fellow Texan, Assistant Surgeon Isaiah J. Roberts, writing to Roberts later that day. The exact topic and outcome of the discussion are unknown—Roberts resigned from the army later in the year because of poor health—but Moore obviously had to balance political expedience with his own sense of propriety. It is likely that the surgeon general was also pressured by members of Congress to grant furloughs, leaves of absence, or discharges for soldier-constituents. If Moore harbored any ill feelings toward Congress, it did not prevent him from offering to assign a medical officer to inoculate its members against smallpox with healthy vaccine matter. The proposal, said government clerk John B. Jones, enlivened the legislative session, but the "honor" was declined.[31]

Moore was not without outspoken opponents in Congress. During deliberations about an 1863 bill for improving the Medical Department, Representative William W. Clark of Georgia said that the department was inefficient and neglectful and should not be rewarded. When another congressman reportedly asked Clark if he "intended to arraign the Surgeon General for want of skill and humanity," the Georgian responded, without naming a specific person, that "if the cap fitted anyone, let him wear it."[32]

Jefferson Davis provided this postwar assessment of Moore: "[He] was not a politician, too honest to yield his convictions to the interested applications of members of congress, he encountered their displeasure, and prejudice, radiating from that center deprived him of the credit due." Although direct evidence is scarce, friction between Moore and Confederate legislators and state politicians may have hampered the surgeon general's efforts to improve the Medical Department and influenced some of his decisions.[33]

Whatever the explanation, various pieces of legislation that would have helped the Medical Department were not enacted. That fact, combined with the obsolescence of army regulations, hindered the department's ability to organize itself for maximum efficiency and accounted, in part, for the confusion surrounding a vital level in its command structure—that of medical director.

3. ❧ Medical Directors

The rudimentary structure that defined the Confederate Medical Department in early 1861 soon proved to be inadequate for the huge scale of the Civil War. That inadequacy was the result of the Confederate army having adopted almost verbatim the prewar regulations and practices of the US Army, which were suited for the contingencies of small-scale actions on the frontier. Whereas prewar regulations specified "the formation by divisions" (groups of two or more brigades) as "the basis of the organization of armies in the field," there were no organized units in prewar America larger than a regiment. The organizational level known as a "corps"—a group of two or more divisions as an element of a larger army—was familiar to American students of the Napoleonic Wars but had not yet been used in American wars. The Civil War presented a sudden need to bring together much larger groups of soldiers than had been gathered in American history, and regulations were slow to catch up with the ad hoc organization of fighting units in the field. For the Medical Department, this meant that command levels between the SGO and surgeons in regiments and hospitals would have to be developed and refined.[1]

Levels of Medical Command in the Field

A vital command tier between the SGO and surgeons serving with regiments or in hospitals was that of medical director. The 1861 Confederate army and Medical Department regulations stated that the medical director of a corps—where "corps" was understood to be a multidivisional unit that itself was an army—was assigned by the War Department or the corps's commander and exercised general control over its hospitals and medical officers. No other levels of medical command were described.[2]

Confusion could result when regulations lagged behind organizational changes, such as the one occurring on March 29, 1862, when the Army of the Mississippi (part of the future Army of Tennessee) was formed by bringing together various units, including two grand divisions (of two divisions

27

each) and the three-division Central Army of Kentucky. When merged as the Army of the Mississippi, those three components were called the First, Second, and Third Corps, each with a medical director. At the time, using the term "corps" to describe a multidivisional group within a larger army— other terms with the same meaning included "wing" and "command"—was consistent with military usage but implied nothing specific about the group's command, since a corps was not yet officially recognized in regulations. On April 11 Surgeon George W. Lawrence, medical director of the Army of the Mississippi's Third Corps, complained to his corps commander, Major General William J. Hardee, that Surgeon Andrew Jackson Foard, medical director of the Army of the Mississippi, had barred him from organizing general or brigade hospitals. Foard's interference, said Lawrence, prevented him from complying with Medical Department regulations, which specified that the medical director of an army corps had general control of hospitals; because of this, Lawrence was resigning. The Army of the Mississippi's commander, General P. G. T. Beauregard, refused to accept the surgeon's resignation, however, saying, "This is no time for officers to resign and quit the service because they cannot carry out their own ideas."[3]

On April 15 Medical Director Foard remarked tersely that Lawrence's complaint was groundless and cited March 26 changes to Medical Department regulations and War Department orders of the same date announcing them. The revised regulations stated that an army corps or department—where a "department" was a geographic region controlled by a commanding general— would have not only a medical director but also medical staff officers at the division and brigade levels; as before, the medical director would have general control of surgeons and hospitals. Lawrence thought that, as medical director of the Third Corps of the Army of the Mississippi, he had such control within his own corps. On the other hand, Foard evidently believed that, in this instance, "army corps" applied to the Army of the Mississippi as a whole and that he had overall control of all hospitals in said army, including those in the Third Corps. Hardee wanted to retain Lawrence's services, so he asked Adjutant and Inspector General Cooper to disapprove the resignation and instead have the surgeon report to him for duty. Cooper referred the matter to Surgeon General Moore, who asked on May 28 that the resignation be accepted, which it was.[4]

The basis of this incident was that the relationship between the medical director of a multicorps army and the medical directors of the individual corps remained unclear. Furthermore, exactly what title properly applied to

Lawrence—and to the other so-called medical directors within the Army of the Mississippi—was in doubt. Lawrence was more than a chief surgeon of division because his charge included more than one division, but the regulations mentioned medical directors for army corps and departments only, and "army corps" could seemingly not refer simultaneously to Hardee's Third Corps and to Beauregard's Army of the Mississippi. (In practice, officers in Lawrence's position continued to be called medical directors; in September 1862 Congress recognized a corps as a group of divisions.) Foard's belief that he controlled all of the hospitals of the Army of the Mississippi was later borne out an August 1862 circular from the SGO: "Should different armies be consolidated under one commander, the Medical Directors of the armies thus absorbed cease to act as such. They must report to, and will be governed by the orders of, the Medical Director of the Commanding General." In apparent response to confusion about whether military commanders or medical directors had ultimate control over general hospitals, the AIGO announced in October 1862 that local commanders had that authority but that general management of the facilities should be left to senior surgeons and medical directors. Local commanders should interfere with that management in special cases only, which should be referred to the department commander.[5]

The March 26 War Department orders announcing the changes in Medical Department regulations also directed that "Medical Officers, heretofore styled Medical Directors," who were not in charge of an army corps or military department should assume another approved title. The improper use of titles clearly exasperated Moore. In a letter to Surgeon Foard about his May 1862 reappointment as medical director of the Army of the Mississippi, Moore remarked, "You are expected to remove the evils of a multiplicity of Directors." The problem apparently persisted, for in November Moore called attention to the fact that "certain medical officers—Chief Surgeons of Division, Senior Surgeons of Brigades, or others of less position—style and sign themselves Medical Directors." Moore instructed legitimate medical directors to take steps to prevent the continuance of this irregularity.[6]

Moore was also irritated by surgeons being appointed or calling themselves assistant medical directors. Medical directors were allowed to have medical officers as assistants, but he maintained that "the term 'Asst Medical Director' has no existence in the Medical Regulations, and its use can give rise only to confusion." After learning that Surgeon Augustine S. Mason had been appointed assistant medical director in Major General Gustavus Smith's command in the Department of North Carolina and Southern Virginia, Moore instructed the medical director of that department to have Mason "sign communications, not as 'Asst Medical Director,' but 'by order of the Medical Director.'" The problem evidently continued to arise elsewhere, for general orders issued by the AIGO in September 1863 again prohibited use of the title.[7]

Among the medical officers appointed to assist medical directors were those placed in charge of general hospitals in specific localities. Surgeon Samuel H. Stout, for example, was placed in charge of hospitals in Chattanooga in March 1862 by the commander of the Western Department. In September Surgeon Peter E. Hines was "charged with the supervision and management of the hospitals in Petersburg [Virginia] and its vicinity" by the medical director for Major General Smith's previous command (the defenses of Richmond). Stout and Hines were not called medical directors, but their charge of general hospitals freed their medical directors from that direct responsibility and presaged the later creation of the position of medical director of hospitals.[8]

Orders and legislation further delineating medical staff officers appeared over the next two years. It had been common practice for generals commanding armies and corps to select their medical director. In February 1863 orders from the AIGO specified that "the senior surgeons of commands entitled to medical directors will be detailed as medical directors for such commands." When the interests of the service demanded otherwise, medical directors now would be recommended by the surgeon general and announced by the AIGO. In March new Medical Department regulations confused the matter by stating that medical directors would be recommended by the surgeon general (with no mention of seniority) and once approved—by whom was not stated—announced by the AIGO. Shortly afterward, on April 4, Surgeon James M. Holloway, assigned to Richmond's General Hospital No. 2, wrote to Surgeon General Moore with a claim that he, as the senior medical officer of the post that included Richmond (the Department of Henrico), was entitled to be its medical director. He was indeed senior to the incumbent medical director, and Moore, perhaps unable to rule whether Holloway should displace the incumbent or if the surgeon general's recommendation was required, referred the matter to the secretary of war, who did not award the directorship to Holloway.[9]

The uncertainty surrounding such appointments is illustrated in the naming of Surgeon John M. Johnson as medical director of Hardee's Corps of the Army of Tennessee. On June 20, 1863, Hardee told Brigadier General William W. Mackall, chief of staff for the Army of Tennessee's commanding general, that he had appointed Johnson and desired official confirmation.

Mackall indicated that the appointment was approved, provided that regulations permitted a corps to have a medical director. (They did, and Johnson was replacing a recently departed corps medical director.) Although there is no evidence that Johnson would have been his choice for the position, Moore acknowledged that the appointment was allowed and recommended that it be approved, even though the surgeon was not the senior medical officer in the command.[10]

Johnson's appointment, however, showed how seniority still mattered to some individuals. Dr. James F. Heustis, chief surgeon of a division in Hardee's Corps, told his division commander, Major General John C. Breckinridge, "I could not serve any longer under the present Med. Director of the Corps [Johnson], who is younger in years, younger in the profession, of little or no reputation that I know of, & younger in the service than I am." Heustis also demonstrated a misunderstanding of the role of staff officers. AIGO general orders of July 1862 stated that, except for aides-de-camp, staff officers—such as medical directors—were assigned to the command, not to the commander, and would not necessarily be reassigned when the commanding general left. In contrast, Heustis told Breckinridge, "When I accepted the appointment of Chief Surgeon of your Division it was to serve with you & not with whomever might succeed you in command."[11]

A key development for medical directors occurred in March 1863 with the issuance of AIGO General Orders No. 28, paragraph 5 of which removed control of general hospitals from medical directors in the field and assigned it to "specially selected" officers who would become known as medical directors of hospitals (and are discussed in more detail below). Medical directors of armies, corps, and departments were not to interfere with medical directors of hospitals with regard to general hospitals.[12]

President Davis, impatient with Congress's inability to create acceptable legislation to improve the general staff, directed the issuance of AIGO general orders in April 1864 indicating the number of staff officers. An army composed of two or more corps would have a medical director, who could have an assistant, and a separate medical inspector. A corps would have a medical director-inspector (a combined role), a division would have a chief surgeon-inspector (another combined role), and a brigade's senior surgeon would serve as brigade surgeon and inspector while retaining his regimental duties. All of those assignments would be made via orders from the AIGO. This made clear that armies and corps were separate organizational tiers and that both were entitled to a medical director. As stated in the August 1862

SGO circular, however, when a corps was incorporated into an army—rather than operating on its own—its medical director was subordinate to the army's medical director. Davis approved a general-staff bill on June 14, 1864, which agreed with the AIGO general orders, specified staff officers' ranks, and authorized the president to make appointments; no appointments were made pursuant to the act.[13]

In its fully developed form, the organization of the Medical Department had multiple levels, starting at the bottom, with surgeons and assistant surgeons of regiments, who submitted reports to the senior surgeon of brigade, who then consolidated and forwarded reports to the chief surgeon of division. Above that officer was the medical director of the corps, and above him was the medical director of the army; above all medical directors of armies was the surgeon general. Regiments or brigades acting independently would bypass the division and corps levels by reporting directly to the medical director of the army or to the surgeon general. Serving with an army's medical director would be a field purveyor (see chapter 5). Medical inspectors at the army level were eventually replaced by inspectors who reported to the surgeon general only (see chapter 4).[14]

In light of medical directors' vital role, Surgeon General Moore must have been gratified that those serving in that capacity included officers—Thomas H. Williams and Lafayette Guild, for example—who had served in the US Army, understood their duties, and appreciated the importance of the various bookkeeping responsibilities of surgeons at all levels of the Medical Department. A medical director who knew his job, however, was not always successful in getting his subordinates to do theirs. Surgeon Williams, medical director of the Army of the Potomac, for example, lamented to Moore in November 1861 that he found it "almost impossible to induce the medical officers of our Volunteer Army" to submit required reports. Surgeon Guild, medical director of the Army of Northern Virginia, reported to Moore in August 1862 on casualties for June, stating also that such information was missing from some of his subordinates and that medical officers in his command "failed to supply themselves with the means necessary for keeping a list of casualties." In their defense, said Guild, was the fact that accurate record keeping was almost impossible because of the army's rapid movements and recent battles.[15]

The surgeon general did not hold medical directors faultless. When A. J. Foard was reappointed to that position for the Army of the Mississippi, Moore reminded him to "keep this office well informed of all matters pertaining to the Med. Dept. of your Command. Med. Directors in some cases have been very derelict." Nevertheless, he was careful to respect medical directors' place in the chain of command. When Lieutenant Colonel John P. Fitzgerald of the Twenty-Third Virginia Regiment (of the Army of Northern Virginia) asked Medical Director of Hospitals William A. Carrington about securing a promotion for Assistant Surgeon J. L. Cannon, Carrington replied that Moore would have to act on the request and would first refer it to the medical director of the Army of Northern Virginia for that officer's opinion. The surgeon general, said Carrington, "would not allow any Medical Director [such as Carrington] to influence him about the affairs of a Department for which he is not responsible, and I cannot approach him about this matter in any way."[16]

Medical directors in the field were vital in enforcing discipline at all levels of the Medical Department and channeling information from regiments, brigades, divisions, corps, and armies to the SGO. They were also the primary conduits through which Surgeon General Moore distributed instructions, typically in the form of circulars. In September 1864 the SGO listed eighteen medical directors of armies and corps, about half of whom were assigned to the Army of Northern Virginia or the Army of Tennessee.[17]

Medical Directors of Hospitals

Paragraph 5 of AIGO General Orders No. 28 (March 12, 1863) stated: "General hospitals will be under the supervision and control of medical directors specially selected for the purpose, and announced as such in orders from this office. Medical directors of armies, army corps and department will not interfere with this arrangement in respect to the general hospitals." Notably absent was any indication of how those officers were to be selected and to whom they would report. The secretary of war intended that medical directors of hospitals report to the surgeon general, but it is unclear whether that was ever announced generally. Confusion started almost immediately. On March 17, AIGO Special Orders No. 65 indicated that Surgeon Carrington would *resume* the duties of medical director of hospitals for the city of Richmond and relieve Surgeon John S. Dorsey Cullen in that role. Carrington had served temporarily as medical director for the Department of North Carolina and Southern Virginia, which included Richmond, before the position of medical director of hospitals existed. Cullen was the current medical director (not medical director of hospitals) for that department. No officer had been appointed as its medical director of hospitals between the creation of that position on March 12 and it being assigned to Carrington on the seventeenth.[18]

The appointment prompted a quick complaint to Secretary of War Seddon from Surgeon General Moore. Although Carrington was assigned as medical director of hospitals, Moore believed that the order was misworded and that its actual intent was to install him as medical director for the Department of North Carolina and Southern Virginia. After all, the latter was the office held by Cullen, whom Carrington was relieving, and the word "resume" seemingly referred to Carrington's former stint as the department's temporary medical director. Consequently, Moore pointed out that he should not have gotten the appointment because the necessary criteria for medical director had not been met: Carrington was neither the senior surgeon of the command nor the subject of his own recommendation. Moore claimed to be the best judge of officers' suitability for special duties, argued that Carrington's appointment was a circumvention of his authority, and asked Seddon to apply his "supervisory control" over the AIGO to revoke the order. Before receiving a response, he also recommended that Virginia and North Carolina each have a single medical director of hospitals. That suggestion was adopted quickly in AIGO special orders that turned over the management of all Virginia's general hospitals to Carrington and all of North Carolina's to Surgeon Edward N. Covey. Moore, anticipating that his complaint would result in Carrington's removal, suggested that Surgeon Thomas C. Madison be appointed to the post for Virginia.[19]

A week after Moore's recommendation of Madison, a convoluted response from Adjutant and Inspector General Cooper stated that the appointment in question was indeed for medical director of hospitals but that orders establishing the position had not indicated who would name such appointees. Cooper explained that irregularities in orders issued by the officer who "had been acting as medical director of hospitals" in Richmond (Cullen) compelled him to quickly fill the position, so he invoked his authority to name Carrington by virtue of his own "rank & position as senior general & chief of staff of the Army." Thus, he ignored the chain of command by failing to refer a matter of medical personnel to Moore and then conflated two distinct positions—medical director and medical director of hospitals. The haughty Cooper claimed, "If the Surgeon General had been as prompt to name a medical director for the general hospitals here . . . as he has been to find fault with my special order 65 [which assigned Carrington] he would, in all probability have had the officer so named by him announced in orders." He added that Moore should have had the courtesy of routing his objections through him, "his superior officer," rather than going to the secretary of war. Although Cooper outranked the surgeon general, the AIGO and the Medical Department were technically at the same level, with both reporting to the secretary of war. Moore, for his part, ended up with Carrington—not the man he would have selected—assuming a job with huge responsibilities: medical director of Richmond's general hospitals. He then suffered the added indignity of seeing Carrington placed in control of all general hospitals in Virginia, a role Moore desired for another officer. His military pride was probably hurt more than the Medical Department, for Carrington seemed to serve capably in his new position through the end of the war. The episode showed that Cooper would not hesitate to wield power over Moore even if the surgeon general seemed to be in the right.[20]

Surgeon Covey, recommended by Moore as medical director of hospitals for North Carolina—and so appointed on April 2, 1863—lasted only a few months in the position. According to North Carolina governor Zebulon B. Vance, various Marylanders and Virginians were in his state "filling the offices which were local and permanent in their character" and "making themselves obnoxious to our people." During a visit with President Davis, he had identified Marylander Covey as one of the most objectionable. But when no corrective action was taken, Vance wrote to Secretary of War Seddon on September 3 to ask that the offenders be replaced by North Carolinians. "I am striving with all my power to apologize for these appointments and to reconcile our people to the Administration," and "to be refused such a small concession . . . fills me with disgust." Covey was relieved on September 15—by whose order is unclear—and replaced with Surgeon Peter E. Hines, a North Carolinian. Surgeon General Moore no doubt recognized the pressure put on the Confederate government by individual states but must nevertheless have regretted that decisions about appointing and relieving medical officers were not always his to make and could be based on factors other than merit.[21]

Carrington's appointment demonstrated that one medical director of hospitals could control facilities that were within the boundaries of more than one military department. Carrington assumed control of all general hospitals in Virginia, whether they were in the Department of North Carolina and Southern Virginia or in the Department of Henrico. He reported to the surgeon general rather than to the commanding generals of those two military administrations. Although Carrington understood the distinctions between field and general hospitals, he had to ask Surgeon General Moore exactly which Virginia hospitals were under his charge. A facility in Jerusalem, Virginia, was considered a general hospital by its staff and townspeople and by Lieutenant General James Longstreet, who commanded the Department of

North Carolina and Southern Virginia. Longstreet's medical director, Surgeon Cullen, thought it qualified as a field hospital and thus fell under his own jurisdiction. Similar differences of opinion existed for other facilities. The need to make such distinctions, of course, would not have existed had the position of medical director of hospitals not been created.[22]

The surgeon general was willing to alter, when necessary, the geographical boundaries over which a medical director of hospitals had control. In September 1863 Moore noted that patients from the Department of East Tennessee were hospitalized at Emory and Henry College and points west. He recommended that control of those hospitals, all in southwestern Virginia, be placed under the control of the medical director of hospitals for the Department of East Tennessee; the AIGO agreed. Thus, in this instance, some Virginia hospitals were not controlled by Medical Director Carrington.[23]

One example of a medical director of hospitals assigned to a specific command was Surgeon Frank A. Ross. In November 1863 Ross was medical director for the Department of the Gulf, commanded by Major General Dabney Maury. Late in the month he was ordered to assume the role of medical director of hospitals for that command, an assignment that would remove him from Maury's authority. Ross asserted that there were so few general hospitals in the region that he would have little to do and charged that Surgeon General Moore knew the situation. Evidently considering the order a demotion, the doctor resigned his commission. Maury called Ross "an intelligent and courteous gentleman whose feelings are naturally wounded by the change which has been made in his position" and regretted that the assignment would deprive him of the surgeon's service. The incident illustrates not only how a surgeon's pride could interfere with Moore's plans but also that Maury and Ross, at least, understood that a medical director of hospitals, responsible for hospitals within a command area, did not answer to its commanding general.[24]

Surgeon Stokes A. Smith, assigned as medical director of hospitals for the Trans-Mississippi Department, had his own ideas about the reporting structure. He believed that the separate districts of the department each needed its own surgeon to take charge of general hospitals. Such officers would be on the staff of the district's commanding general and report to both the district's medical director and to Smith. By the time he offered this view, in late August 1863, the Trans-Mississippi Department—isolated because of Federal control of the Mississippi River—was essentially operating as its own entity, separate from the government in Richmond. Yet his interpretation seemed to contradict the provision of General Orders No. 28, that medical directors of armies, corps, and departments were not to interfere with the functions of medical directors of hospitals.[25]

Meanwhile, the aforementioned Surgeon Heustis of the Army of Tennessee, upon learning of the new position of medical director of hospitals, on April 18, 1863, expressed his wish to receive that title and be assigned to duty at Mobile for reasons related to the health and welfare of his family. Lieutenant General Hardee, his corps commander, disapproved the application on the grounds that Heustis, as chief surgeon of division, would be difficult to replace and had based his request "on personal considerations alone." Because of the absence of an official explanation of how appointments to those positions were to be made, it is unclear whether Hardee had the authority to block the doctor's application. In September 1864 an official announcement showed Heustis being stationed in Mobile and having two positions—medical director and medical director of hospitals—that were not intended to be held by the same individual.[26]

Commanders' Attempt to Retain Control of General Hospitals

The creation of medical directors of hospitals caused anxiety for Surgeon Samuel H. Stout of the Army of Tennessee. Stout had been appointed superintendent of hospitals by General Bragg in mid-1862 and reported to the army's medical director. Although his title was unrecognized in regulations, the appointment was legitimate in that Stout could be considered an assistant to the medical director. The AIGO's creation of the position of medical director of hospitals now caused him to worry that a new appointee would displace him, and it raised concerns in Bragg, who wanted to retain control of general hospitals in his command through his medical director. A number of preemptive appeals on Stout's behalf were sent to Surgeon General Moore, but AIGO special orders announced first, on April 23, 1863, that Surgeon Lewis T. Pim was appointed medical director of general hospitals of Bragg's army and then, on May 14, that Stout was appointed inspector of the same hospitals. Further exchanges involving Bragg resulted in the earlier assignments being revoked and Stout being named medical director of hospitals.[27]

Stout considered Bragg's creation of a superintendent of hospitals to be a stroke of genius in relieving from his medical director the burden of directly administering the hospitals while retaining the general's overall control of those facilities through that officer. The War Department, said Stout, saw the wisdom of Bragg's action and emulated it in the creation of medical directors of hospitals. He maintained that Surgeon General Moore overestimated his own ability to control distant general hospitals from Richmond and had never considered creating a position similar to his own. In these assertions, Stout was largely in error. Although the order establishing medical directors of hospitals omitted any mention of reporting structure, the intent was for those officers to report to the surgeon general, not to local commanding generals. In addition, the War Department, far from using Bragg's appointment as a model, demonstrated its ignorance of the superintendent's role when it named Surgeon Pim to assume duties that Stout was already performing. A letter from Surgeon General Moore to Surgeon Foard added important context. Foard had reported that General Bragg wanted to maintain the status quo of having his general hospitals under the control of his medical director. Moore replied, "This matter has been regulated by the Sec War and is therefore beyond the control of this Bureau [the SGO]." Furthermore, he said, "It is proper to remark that this office had no knowledge directly or indirectly of [the order] creating Medical Directors of hospitals, until it was published." The surgeon general may have had a role in creating medical directors of hospitals, but it appears that the president, secretary of war, or AIGO launched the position without telling him.[28]

Bragg was not alone in his desire to keep general hospitals under local control. Lieutenant General Leonidas Polk, one of his corps commanders, told Adjutant and Inspector General Cooper that the establishment of medical directors of hospitals was "not expedient or wise" and that the general hospitals of a corps should be controlled by that corps's medical director. The concerns of these generals may have been unfounded, since Surgeon Stout found that his transition to medical director of hospitals for the Army of Tennessee did not alter his relationship with Bragg and was beneficial in putting himself in more direct communication with the surgeon general.[29]

Major General J. E. B. Stuart, cavalry commander with the Army of Northern Virginia, and his division surgeon, Talcott Eliason, also appeared desirous of controlling their own general hospitals when they proposed establishing multiple "small hospitals throughout the country" rather than sending their sick and wounded to the large general facilities in Richmond. That army's medical director, Surgeon Guild, countered by outlining the problems with their plan. First, the proposed hospitals would require additional medical officers, other personnel, and materials. Second, "when a sudden or rapid movement of the army is made it is next to an impossibility to break up the small hospitals . . . and the inmates are consequently paroled by the enemy." Eliason had evidently suggested a location for a division hospital, and Guild offered to approve the establishment of a general hospital there instead if it did not present the problems he had mentioned. Stuart subsequently dispatched Eliason to Richmond "on business connected with the establishment of a General Hospital for the Cav. Div."[30]

General Joseph E. Johnston evidently tried to keep general hospitals under his control as commander of the Department of Mississippi. In November 1863 Moore complained to Cooper that Johnston had begun converting permanent, fixed hospitals far removed from his troops' area of operations (that is, general hospitals) into field hospitals by naming the facilities after corps, divisions, and brigades in his army. He objected to the general's "arbitrary application of terms, and the consequent disarrangement of the general plan of organization, heretofore successfully adopted, and the accompanying disadvantages of the system he has inaugurated." Moore argued that "two years of experience have fully shown, how utterly impossible it is, for the ablest Medical Directors, serving with Troops in the Field, to bestow upon hospitals in the rear, that care and attention so essential to their efficiency and usefulness." Thus, although having previously denied advance knowledge of the order that established medical directors of hospitals, he supported the rationale behind the position.[31]

Administrative Confusion about Medical Directors of Hospitals

A final example illustrates the confusion at various levels about medical directors of hospitals. On July 17, 1863, Moore told Cooper that two hospital surgeons had each been granted a sixty-day leave of absence by the headquarters of the Department of South Carolina and Georgia. "This, it is believed," the surgeon general noted tersely, "is in violation of Regulations & General Orders." The AIGO, responding for the secretary of war, told General Beauregard, commander of the Department of South Carolina and Georgia, that hospital surgeons were subordinate to the medical director of hospitals—in Beauregard's command, that office was filled by Surgeon Nathaniel S. Crowell— who, in turn, was subordinate to the surgeon general. (In other words, Beauregard was not authorized to grant the leaves.) The exasperated general replied: "That a Medical Director [Crowell] should be ordered to report to me for duty with Hospitals over which I have no control . . . I must respectfully say, is hardly to be expected. . . . Have I command over [Crowell]—if not why should [he] report to me for assignment?—if so, can it be that I do not Command those who are under this Command!" When this made its way back to the SGO, Moore remarked that his intent was actually to point out that regulations required that applications for a leave of longer than thirty days were to be referred to the secretary of war for a decision. The exchange—which would have been shorter had Moore been more explanatory in his original communication—not only demonstrated ignorance of regulations (regarding leaves of absence) on the part of Beauregard, the secretary of war, and the AIGO but also raised the issue of reporting. Was a medical director of hospitals responsible to the surgeon general, as maintained by the secretary of war, or to the commander of the military department to which that director was assigned, as assumed by Beauregard? That point was not resolved, but it is tempting to believe that Moore derived some satisfaction from showing that his superiors, who had bypassed him when making key decisions about his own department, knew less about regulations than he did.[32]

A September 1864 list from the SGO indicated eight medical directors of hospitals. In some cases the areas of responsibility for those officers were expressed in geographical terms. Virginia and North Carolina, for example, were each covered by one appointee. Other medical directors of hospitals were assigned to specific military commands and were to present themselves to the department's or army's commanding general, at least when first reporting for duty. Even if the assigned geographical region and the area controlled by a military command were identical, the question of reporting remained. Medical directors of commands were not to interfere with medical directors of hospitals, but if the latter were responsible to commanding generals, then medical directors might exert influence through those officers.[33]

The vague description of the position of medical director of hospitals confused individuals who sought, were appointed, or had the fortune to be the hierarchal superior to that office. The situation was not improved by the apparent exclusion of the surgeon general in describing and announcing the position.

The size and evolving organization of the Confederate army made preexisting regulations and practices inadequate for defining the organizational standing and responsibilities of medical directors. The same held true for another group of officers under the surgeon general's command—medical inspectors.

4. ✤ Medical Inspectors

Samuel Preston Moore recognized almost immediately upon being named acting surgeon general that the vast influx of inexperienced military personnel, including those assigned to the Medical Department, could seriously impair efforts to improve and maintain the health of the army. As a career military surgeon, he well realized the importance of discipline in enforcing regulations concerning cleanliness, proper nutrition, and other factors that promoted good health in hospitals and camps, observing in early 1862:

> Whatever differences of opinion may exist among enlightened men, as to the extent to which disease may be successfully opposed when it has invaded the human system, there is unanimity as to the efficiency of measures of prevention, when clearly discerned and rigidly enforced. . . . It must be admitted that an intelligent and authoritative supervision over matters pertaining to the hygiene of the army is demanded. Serious as are the responsibilities of the Medical man; and fatal as are the consequences where those responsibilities are not duly appreciated; it is a lamentable fact that there is a strong tendency to forget the disastrous results that flow from neglect or an unintelligent routine in the discharge of duty.[1]

Moore thought that medical inspectors would help detect deleterious practices and promote hygienic conditions, but he did not have an abundance of qualified personnel to dedicate to such posts. According to regulations, a hospital's chief surgeon was responsible for regular inspections of his own facility, and medical directors had responsibility for inspection of hospitals in their command. There were no provisions, however, for separate medical inspectors, and there was no clarity about where surgeons' inspections reports were to be sent. A congressional committee recommended that the reports be sent to the commander to whose staff the inspecting surgeon was attached and also to the army's inspector general. The inspector general was charged with determining whether army regulations were properly carried out. In the Confederate army the offices of adjutant general and inspector general were combined (thus the AIGO), a situation that left inadequate time for the hybrid organization to conduct its own inspections of army facilities, including hospitals.[2]

Early Appointment of Inspectors

As if in recognition of its own inability to carry out inspections, the AIGO on August 7, 1861, ordered that to Surgeon Lafayette Guild, "having been appointed 'Inspector of Hospitals,' the chiefs of the different staff departments will afford him every possible facility in the discharge of his duties: when any immediate change of arrangements with regard to the sick may become necessary, the suggestions of Surg. Guild will be carried out, without reference to these Head Quarters [AIGO]." The impetus behind that order is unknown but was probably came from Moore; the initial order assigning Guild, a former US Army surgeon, to the position and describing his duties remains lost. In any event, the August 7 order is remarkable in the authority granted to Guild and in the cooperation demanded from the chiefs of the Quartermaster and Subsistence Departments. Guild's tenure as inspector of hospitals appears to have been short since he was given other inspection duties a few months later.[3]

As a result of this, on September 12 Moore took the expedient measure of instructing medical directors to urge their commanding general to designate a surgeon or assistant surgeon to conduct inspections. He told them that the selected individual would "make from time to time . . . a thorough inspection of Hospitals subject to your control, as well as of the sick in the field" and report to the medical director "all facts coming within his reach, the knowledge of which, may lead to the better care and protection of our sick and wounded; at the same time suggesting as his judgement may prompt, any measures of hygiene calculated to diminish the amount of sickness now so prevalent in our camp." Moore expected the commanding general to facilitate the performance of the inspector's mission. He probably envisioned the selected individual retaining his responsibilities as a regimental surgeon, an arrangement that bypassed the necessity to provide an additional medical officer to the command. Yet it might be problematic for an inspecting officer to report shortcomings attributable to the neglect or misbehavior of surgeons in his own command, some of whom might outrank him. Moore, in fact, refrained from describing the inspectors' duties as reporting on or addressing corrective measures to individual surgeons. He did not indicate that the designated officers were to be called "medical inspectors," so it is unlikely that they were given that title (the lack of which makes it difficult to identify men who served in this role).[4]

The surgeon general's directive was followed in January 1862 by a recommendation of a special congressional committee that inspectors be added to the medical staff. Problems with the army's health, comfort, and efficiency, declared the committee, stemmed largely from regulations not being enforced and from the lack of a regular system of inspections. Using that report as a springboard, Moore recommended legislation that called for the appointment of medical inspectors, each having the rank and allowance of a surgeon with two years of service, one of whom would be assigned to each military district and report to him. Among the aims of the new inspectors would be "the securing of a more rigid accountability as to the discharge of duty, by Regimental Medical Officers, and Surgeons and Assistant Surgeons of Hospitals." Giving inspectors adequate rank and separating them from the reporting hierarchy of the commands they were reviewing were meant to ensure necessary cooperation from other officers and remove the awkwardness of inspectors criticizing colleagues in their own command. The House bill resulting from the committee's report and Moore's recommendation, however, died in the Senate in April.[5]

A subsequent bill that called for medical inspectors was vetoed by President Davis in October, despite general agreement about the need for inspectors. On being asked his view of the measure, Surgeon Edwin S. Gaillard noted that "nothing . . . would tend, as much as this course of action [organizing a corps of inspectors], to increase the safety and welfare of our sick and to promote the efficiency and vitality of the Medical Department." He also agreed with the rationale for conferring adequate rank on inspectors: "As these officers will be detached from field and hospital duty, exercising no conferred authority from a General, in the field acting for the most part independently, it will be of course necessary, that, to ensure obedience on the part of Regimental and other officers in the Department, that there should be increased rank conferred."[6]

Moving toward Central Assignment of Inspectors

As with other aspects of the Medical Department, the reporting structure for medical inspectors became more centralized over time, with inspectors reporting less to local commanding officers and more to the surgeon general himself.

The aforementioned congressional committee had noted that medical directors, although charged with inspecting their own hospitals, often lacked the time to do so. Medical directors seemed to agree with this and, because they were allowed to have assistants, appointed their own medical inspectors from among their regimental surgeons or suggested other officers whom their commanding generals added to their general staff in that capacity. Since they were responsible to their medical director, however, those inspectors still faced the possibility of having to report the deficiencies of surgeons in their own command. That problem was neatly expressed in September shortly after Surgeon Gaillard became medical director of the Department of North Carolina and Southern Virginia. Gaillard approached Surgeon St. George Tucker Peachy about being inspector of hospitals for Richmond. Peachy, who had held that position in late 1861, claimed poor health but stated two other reasons for declining the post: "In the first place the position is a thankless one and in it one gains nothing but enemies. It is impossible to do otherwise. Secondly my personal relations with some surgeons in charge of hospitals would cause any unfavorable report I might deem proper to make to you to be attributed to personal spleen and ire on my part vented upon them from behind the impregnable defence of *officiality*."[7]

Moore, determined to have a group of medical inspectors who would report directly to him, evidently obtained War Department approval to start naming, through the AIGO, a small number of trusted officers to such roles. Thus, in December 1861 the AIGO ordered Surgeon Guild to inspect the hospital and camps of the commands of Generals Lee and Bragg and the "hospitals and camps of instruction contiguous thereto." He was to make a full report of his findings directly to the surgeon general. During the same month, Surgeon William W. Anderson was ordered to inspect camps, hospitals, and the offices of the medical purveyor and medical director in the Western Department; he was to receive special instructions directly from Moore. Then in mid-1862 Surgeons Thomas C. Madison and Thomas H. Williams were ordered to inspect general hospitals in specific geographic areas. Guild, Anderson, Madison, and Williams were apt choices because their previous service as US Army surgeons made them familiar with regulations and with the importance of discipline. In April 1863 another trusted officer, Surgeon Gaillard, joined the group of inspectors reporting to Moore. The specific assignments for those officers were changed from time to time.[8]

Moore's desire to control medical inspectors was further gratified by an AIGO general order in September 1863 that read, "Medical inspectors will be recommended by the Surgeon General, and being approved, will be announced in orders from this office [the AIGO]." Moore took two immediate steps. First, he began assigning inspectors to examine the field hospitals and camps of various commands, including the Army of Northern Virginia, the Department of North Carolina, and the Department of South Carolina, Georgia, and Florida. Second, he informed medical directors of the AIGO order and specified that any current medical inspector not so announced by the office should submit to the SGO a copy of the order assigning him to that position along with remarks or recommendations of the medical director. The response was apparently unsatisfactory, for four months later, in January 1864, Moore informed medical directors that medical inspectors for army corps, divisions, and brigades were being assigned in violation of the AIGO order—that is, without his recommendation and AIGO approval. Properly assigned medical inspectors, the surgeon general stated, were not to be included in the returns of medical officers they submitted; that stipulation emphasized that field medical inspectors were not to be part of a command's general staff but instead were to report directly to the SGO. If a properly assigned inspector was needed where one did not already exist, that circumstance was to be reported to the SGO.[9]

President Davis confused matters by having the AIGO issue special orders in April 1864 regarding the number of officers allowed on the general staff of army commands. An army was allowed a medical inspector (separate from its medical director), while corps, divisions, and brigades each were allowed a chief medical officer—called the medical director, chief surgeon, and brigade surgeon, respectively—who would also serve as medical inspector. Officers filling those posts were to be assigned by the AIGO. In allowing medical inspectors as members of the general staff, the orders seemed to contradict its general order of September 1863 that—at least as Moore interpreted it—separated medical inspectors from the general staff.[10]

By September 1864 the Medical Department had seven medical inspectors of general hospitals and six medical inspectors of field hospitals and camps; two of the latter had the special assignment of superintending the vaccination (against smallpox) of troops in the armies, hospitals, and camps of instruction. The surgeon general also assigned officers to inspect medical-purveying depots. Additional surgeons were ordered, late in the war, to inspect hospitals, though not with the purpose of improving medical care. Instead, their purpose was to "return to the field all detailed men and patients fit for duty."[11]

Additional Inspectors

Hospital inspections were also carried out on behalf of the AIGO. For example, Lieutenant Colonel John S. Saunders, an artillery officer, submitted reports to Cooper's office for eight Richmond-area hospitals that he had inspected in late 1864 and early 1865. In February 1865 Surgeon William A. Carrington, in charge of Virginia's general hospital, requested the names of those individuals authorized to inspect the state's hospitals. He was told that all officers on general AIGO inspection duty were so authorized, although none were specifically instructed to inspect hospitals.[12]

Some consideration was given to expanding the number of medical inspectors of hospitals late in the war. In January 1865 Surgeon General Moore told Congressman David Clopton, chairman of the House Standing Committee on the Medical Department, that additional officers were unnecessary. In doing so he described how hospitals were currently inspected:

> Medical Inspectors of *Hospitals* . . . are now assigned to duty in orders by the Adjt & Insp General, on the recommendation of this Office. . . . In order that these Inspectors may not become subjected to local influences, the respective spheres of their Inspections are, from time to time, changed.
>
> They are required to inspect thoroughly each hospital in their districts, once in each month, and to make, to this Office monthly a full and minute report of their Inspections. . . . These Inspections are regularly, and, I am satisfied, faithfully made. . . . These Reports are rigidly examined and all errors, neglects and irregularities therein reported are referred . . . to the Chief of the Departments in which such errors, neglects or irregularities may exist. For the correction of those found in this Department, instructions are issued, remedies suggested, and negligent and inefficient or unfaithful officers promptly censured, or relieved and sent to the field. It is believed that this system operates well, and its fruits are apparent in a generally improved condition and administration.
>
> Besides these Inspectors, efficient and reliable medical officers are sent to investigate and make special report, whenever special grievances or mismanagement of any character is reported.
>
> In the interior administration of Hospitals, a daily inspection and minute Report . . . is made by the officer of the day, and the following

Inspections required from the other medical officers of the Hospital, viz: A general inspection of all the Hospitals under his charge, on the last day of each month by the Surgeon in Charge of Hospitals. A general inspection every Sunday morning at 9 A.M. by the Senior Surgeon of each special Hospital or Hospital Division.

Still other Inspections are made by officers of the Adjt & Insp Genl's Department, and other officers upon the Staffs of Generals. The result of these latter Inspections, often conducted by those not all conversant with hospital administration, or the regulations by which it is controlled, are seldom received at this Office. Their number and frequency are reported by faithful medical officers, as an embarrassment to them in the full performance of their duties, and it is hoped that Congress will not consider it necessary to further authorize this unnecessary system, by legal enactment.

Why members of Congress thought that additional inspectors were needed is unclear. Also unknown is why Moore objected to having more positions authorized. Perhaps he believed that the additional positions would be filled regardless and deprive him of useful surgeons who could be assigned elsewhere.[13]

The surgeon general maintained personnel in Richmond who had responsibilities related to inspections. Surgeon Gaillard, assigned to examine general hospitals in various parts of Virginia, was directed to base himself in Richmond; his office was a short walk from the Mechanics Institute, where the SGO was established. Surgeon Francis Sorrel, in addition to being inspector of hospitals for Richmond, was considered by Moore to be an "absolutely indispensable" member of his staff. Surgeon Herman Baer, also considered absolutely indispensable by the surgeon general, worked in the SGO and examined inspection reports. In addition, soldiers detailed to the SGO as clerks examined inspection reports.[14]

Using medical inspectors to optimize healthful conditions was accomplished through Surgeon General Moore's initiative with some assistance from the AIGO. His leadership was also apparent in the system organized to equip his surgeons with sufficient medicines and other supplies—medical purveying.

5. Medical Purveyors

Medical purveyors—surgeons who procured and distributed drugs and other medical supplies—were vital in efforts to care for the sick and wounded and to prevent disease. As was the case with medical directors and medical inspectors, the Medical Department's approach to organizing purveyors' assignments and duties evolved as officials began to recognize the possible scale and length of the war. (The actual procurement of medical supplies is described in chapters 6 and 7.)

The importance of purveyors is illustrated by the fact that Surgeon David Camden DeLeon was ordered to proceed to New Orleans as medical director and medical purveyor for the Military District of Louisiana on April 22, 1861, more than two weeks before he was appointed acting surgeon general. It was common for medical directors named early in the war to assume the responsibilities, if not the official additional title, of medical purveyor. Surgeon John M. Haden, who succeeded DeLeon in New Orleans, held both titles, as did Surgeons Henry P. Howard and Elisha P. Langworthy in the Department of Texas, Surgeons Alexander N. Talley and Robert A. Kinloch in the Department of South Carolina, and Surgeon Richard Potts in Department No. 2. The 1861 Confederate Medical Department regulations defined their role: "The *Medical Purveyors* [original emphasis] will, under the direction of the Surgeon General, purchase all medical and hospital supplies required for the medical department of the army."[1]

Over the first several months of the war, it became apparent that medical directors needed separate officers appointed as purveyors and, later, that their numbers would have to grow. On October 30, 1861, for example, Surgeon Kinloch was ordered to replace Surgeon Talley at Charleston as medical director and medical purveyor. Shortly thereafter, on November 19, Surgeon J. J. Chisolm, who was acting medical director at Charleston for a short time before Kinloch took command, began serving as medical purveyor. Chisolm was responsible for supplying troops for a large area—South Carolina, Georgia, and eastern Florida—and the topic of having a separate purveyor for Georgia was discussed by early December. On February 28, 1862, he suggested to Surgeon General Moore the possibility of having purveyors stationed at Savannah and Tallahassee. On March 10 Assistant Surgeon William H. Prioleau, who had assisted Medical Directors Talley and Kinloch at Charleston, was assigned as medical purveyor at Savannah. Such actions anticipated the Medical Department regulations of April 10, which specified that purveyors were to be assigned to army corps or military departments.[2]

E. W. Johns as "Chief Purveyor"

One notable exception to the early practice of assigning a single officer as both a medical director and purveyor was Surgeon Edward W. Johns, who was assigned on June 5, 1861, as medical purveyor for Richmond. Johns's responsibilities were expanded in early 1862 in concert with a one-letter change in regulations. Whereas the previous year's regulations defined the role of "medical purveyors," the army regulations of March 13, 1862, paragraph 1156, contained identical wording except for inexplicably assigning that role to the "medical purveyor" (singular). On April 7, at the request of Surgeon General Moore, AIGO Special Orders No. 79 announced that Johns was "recognized as the Medical Purveyor referred to in Paragraph 1156, Army Regulations," and that other medical purveyors were to obey all instructions issued by him "relative to the transfer of medical supplies, and reports of supplies on hand." (The plural "purveyors" was restored in the 1863 army regulations.) Johns's standing was amended the next day in special orders that directed purveyors to obey the same types of instructions coming from Johns but no longer recognized him as "*the* Medical Purveyor." Instead, he was identified simply as "Surgeon E. W. Johns, Medical Purveyor at the principal purveying depot [Richmond]." Johns's newly announced duties—issuing orders about the transfer and inventory of supplies—were narrow and implied no decision-making role in how those supplies were procured. Moore probably intended to make many of those decisions himself.[3]

Johns immediately began issuing circulars to medical purveyors and signing himself as "Chief Purveyor." Among the most informative were Circular No. 1, issued on April 12, 1862, and No. 3, which superseded No. 1 on April 25. Those communications outlined the duties of depot and field purveyors and established nine geographic districts (not necessarily aligned with military districts), each to be supplied by a depot commanded by a depot purveyor. Regimental and hospital medical officers were to route their requisitions for medical supplies upward through the chain of command to their medical director and thence to the field purveyor of the army corps for fulfilment. Field purveyors could purchase supplies locally or replenish their stock by requisitions sent through Johns's office to the nearest depot purveyor, who was chiefly responsible for the purchase of those supplies; the circulars named commanders for most of the depots. Supplies for which depot purveyors were responsible included not only medicines and surgical instruments but also practically all material items needed in a field or general hospital (for example, cots, bedclothes, basins, pitchers, chamber pots, and such). Since goods purchased in bulk had to be repackaged, they also had to obtain the supplies (for example, bottles, tins, labels, and so on) to make that possible.[4]

Johns's Richmond office and warehouses were on Fourteenth Street (also called Pearl Street) between Main and Cary Streets, about six blocks from the SGO. But unlike Richmond medical inspector Francis Sorrel, whose office was also in a building separated from the SGO, Johns was not considered part of Surgeon General Moore's staff. According to one observer in 1864, he had been directing an extemporized subdepartment of the Medical Department, the formation of which had become necessary because the surgeon general's attention could not be diverted from the department's "professional duties." Although Johns did in fact direct other purveyors in the movement and inventory of supplies—this while still operating as purveyor for Richmond—he was not independent of Moore, especially when indigenous remedies, a particular interest of the surgeon general's, were concerned. Johns's dual responsibilities led to awkward situations. For example, although he instructed Surgeon Chisolm, medical purveyor at Charleston, about obtaining and transferring medical goods, he also ordered supplies from him for his own depot in Richmond. When Chisolm sent those items, he routinely instructed Johns to submit the proper receipt paperwork to him and to the surgeon general, as was required by regulations.[5]

Johns's referring to himself as chief purveyor caused confusion. Assistant Surgeon Prioleau, depot purveyor at Savannah and Macon, routinely included that title in letters to Johns. Johns forwarded one such communication, in August 1862, to the surgeon general in response to a query. Moore, before answering the question, corrected Prioleau by informing him "that the Regulations recognize no such title as Chief Purveyor." On September 5 Johns, again signing himself as chief purveyor, ordered Prioleau to immediately send a large portion of his stock to another depot, an action that would make it difficult for him to supply troops in his own region. Prioleau, recalling Moore's correction, surmised that if Johns's title was invalid, he was no longer to be obeyed. He thus declined to follow this order and telegraphed Moore on September 8 for guidance. Moore replied that the nonexistence of the title of chief purveyor did not cancel the earlier directive to obey Johns's orders. His own objection to the unofficial title mirrored his irritation with other medical officers taking on titles not found in regulations. In fact, by September 11 Johns— probably under instructions from Moore—stopped calling himself chief purveyor and substituted "Surgeon and Medical Purveyor." It is unclear whether other purveyors noticed the change, for Surgeon Chisolm kept addressing Johns as chief purveyor until at least early November. The surgeon general could easily have prevented the misunderstanding by telling Prioleau why he was correcting him and what effect, if any, the correction had on Johns's authority. On the other hand, it was not his style to say more than was needed at the moment or to address the implications of his statements. The incident does raise the question of whether Moore saw Johns as being desirous of higher rank and a prestigious title.[6]

At some undetermined time before late February 1863, President Davis received a paper—he did not disclose its originator—that he described as a "project of a bill" proposing the formation of a purveyor general's office as a new component of the army's general staff, separate from the Medical Department and headed by a purveyor general with the rank of colonel. The new office, said the document, was needed because the current "purveying department" (Johns and the purveyors he directed) was concerned entirely with supply, like the Quartermaster or Subsistence Departments, and had nothing to do with the "professional" functions of the Medical Department. Furthermore, the surgeon general could not properly attend to the professional and supply functions of the Medical Department at the same time, and Johns did not have adequate authority over purveyors as long as Moore, his superior, could interfere. Davis put the document aside until he was reminded of it by AIGO general orders issued on February 25, prompted a month earlier by a request from Moore, that relieved Johns from duties he had performed as so-called chief purveyor and transferred them to Moore; Johns retained his responsibilities as purveyor for Richmond. The president had evidently been considering legislation regarding medical purveyors, for he told Secretary of War Seddon that the aforesaid document was not exactly what he had in mind but deserved his consideration. Davis also feared "unfortunate consequences" stemming from the February 25 order and asked Seddon to reconsider it.[7]

The most likely explanation for these events is that Johns or an ally, on learning that legislation about purveyors was being contemplated, created the document to set the stage for elevating Johns to the new position of purveyor general. Moore was almost certainly not the proposal's originator, given that it painted him as a meddling administrator incapable of handling all his responsibilities and placed Johns at a level equal to his own. Although he evidently favored assigning a surgeon to direct purveying operations, Moore wanted that officer in his department and seemed not to accept the notion that the supply functions of purveyors were distinct from and unrelated to the professional duties of medical officers. The surgeon general—whether aware of the "project of a bill" or not—may have either wanted Johns removed as a threat to his authority or been convinced that no single officer could effectively oversee the movement and inventory of medical supplies for the entire army and direct his own large purveying depot at the same time, as Johns was then assigned. The fact that Davis asked Seddon to reconsider the order removing some of Johns's authority indicates that the topic was important enough to draw the president's attention and that the secretary of war probably agreed with Moore about the order's issuance. Announcing the reduction of Johns's authority in AIGO general orders—rather than in special orders—seems heavy handed on the part of Adjutant and Inspector General Cooper but may simply have been a convenience since another paragraph in the general orders dealt with medical directors.[8]

Return of Command to the SGO

Johns's former responsibilities regarding the movement and inventory of supplies officially reverted back to Moore but were at some point assigned, at least in part, to Surgeon Thomas H. Williams as "assistant in charge of purveying business of the Medical Bureau." Williams was ordered to join the SGO on January 14, 1863, perhaps for the surgeon general to have him in place to assume the responsibilities that were shortly to be stripped from Johns. He had served as a medical director and inspector and seems to have earned Moore's confidence. As director of purveying, Williams was considered part of the SGO, but details about his performance in that role remain unavailable. There appear to have been no important changes in the administration of medical purveying after he arrived at the SGO.[9]

President Davis's desire for legislation concerning medical purveyors prompted the introduction of Senate Bill S. 80 on March 12, 1863. Among its provisions were the formation of a corps of medical purveyors, consisting of a purveyor general, two assistant purveyors general, and up to ten purveyors—with the assimilated rank of lieutenant colonel, major, and captain, respectively—all under control of the surgeon general. The bill passed the Senate but not the House.[10]

Depot Purveyors and Their Districts

The nine purveying districts indicated by Johns in his Circular No. 3 had their respective depots located in Richmond, Charlotte, Charleston, Savannah, Atlanta, Montgomery, Jackson, New Orleans, and San Antonio. The single-most-active district, with respect to dealing directly with importers, included the ports of Wilmington and Charleston and was directed by Surgeon and Medical Purveyor Chisolm. At least two additional depots—in Wytheville, Virginia, and in Mobile—were established at about the same time. Surgeons not originally named as depot purveyors appear to have created them, and these sites served as major stationary depots throughout most of the war, even if they were not the sole providers for the purveying districts in which they were located. Surgeon Robinson Miller, for example, directed the Mobile depot even though one existed in Montgomery, the city named in Circular No. 3 as the depot site for Purveying District 6 (Alabama). Miller also served as surgeon in charge of a general hospital in Mobile while directing the depot there.[11]

Depot purveyors were meant to report to Johns or the surgeon general only, an intention not entirely realized in the case of Surgeon Potts. When Johns issued Circular No. 3 in April 1862, Potts was medical director and medical purveyor for the Western Department (also known as Department No. 2) and stationed at Jackson, Mississippi. It named Potts as the depot purveyor for Purveying District 7, which encompassed Mississippi, western Tennessee, and Arkansas. It is unclear whether Potts at that time was officially relieved of his staff duties, for he continued to be associated with various military commands and found himself ordered from place to place, not always at the direction of Johns or Surgeon General Moore. In January 1864, for example, Acting Medical Director Preston B. Scott of the Department of Alabama, Mississippi, and East Florida referred to Potts as the "Depot Med Purveyor for this Department" and recommended that he be ordered to move his supplies to Montgomery.[12] In July Major General Maury, commander of that department, ordered Potts to move his supplies from Montgomery to Mobile.

When informed of the order, the surgeon general asked the AIGO to correct Maury's view of Potts's position:

> As Surg. Potts is a *Depot* Purveyor, he is not subject to orders from Comdg. Generals. As there is already a Purveyor at Mobile, it is not understood why Surg. Potts should be directed to move his depot to that point. These Medical Officers are assigned to certain Posts for performance of specific duties, viz. the supplying of certain Hospitals and Districts. And if they are to move their supplies by order of Comdg. Genls. (except in cases when from movements of the enemy they may be in danger of capture), the arrangements made by this Bureau can never be permanent, and always liable to be broken up and much suffering may be caused to the sick and wounded of the Army.[13]

The AIGO referred the matter to Secretary of War Seddon, who upheld Moore's position. In response Maury again called Potts the purveyor for his department, stated that he was following the surgeon's recommendation to relocate to Mobile, and mentioned that Moore had previously stationed him at Mobile. (Potts's previous move to Mobile was in response to the capture of Jackson, where he had been stationed.) Perhaps Potts had not clearly understood his place in the command structure. The surgeon general's final comment in the exchange about Maury's order was to Potts: "When any change of station is desired, this office should be consulted & not Dept. Commanders."[14]

Moore responded vigorously to perceived encroachments on purveying depots by high-ranking officers. Medical Purveyor Prioleau informed him in July 1864 that General Bragg—at the time military advisor to President Davis—had ordered men detailed to Prioleau's Macon depot to report to the Army of Tennessee. Moore complained to Secretary of War Seddon that the affected soldiers were vital to the operation of the depot, which itself was critically important in supplying Georgia hospitals and the Army of Tennessee. He also noted that most of the men, who had been detailed to Macon by Seddon's orders, were physically disabled and that their original units were now in another army (the Army of Northern Virginia). Moore closed by asking for their immediate return and an explanation of whether Bragg was authorized to override orders of the secretary of war. Seddon referred the matter to Davis. The action attributed to Bragg had evidently derived from Major General Howell Cobb, commander of reserve forces in Georgia, whose orders (according to Davis) had been "to use the powers to call out detailed men . . . as not to embarrass the administrative functions while increasing the powers for defence." The president suggested that Cobb be reminded of those instructions, but it is unclear whether Prioleau got his men back.[15]

In August 1864 Medical Purveyor Miller in Mobile informed Moore that the Quartermaster Department had seized a supply of tin that had been imported by the Medical Department for the manufacture of items for use by hospitals and field infirmaries. Brigadier General Edward Higgins, in charge of bay and harbor defenses at Mobile, had confiscated the tin because it was needed for torpedoes (underwater mines). Surgeon General Moore informed Adjutant and Inspector General Cooper, noting that "the Engineer Bureau enjoys the same facilities for importing its supplies as the Medical Bureau" and asking that the tin be returned. Higgins was immediately ordered to do so.[16]

Since supplies were not equally available in all purveying districts, depot purveyors sent items to each other at the direction of Johns or Moore. The circumstances of war prompted changes in the location of purveying depots, some of which occurred soon after the issuance of Johns's Circular No. 3. The imminent Union capture of New Orleans in late April 1862, for example, forced a Confederate military evacuation of that city; whether the purveying depot there was relocated is unclear. Concerns about other Union advances spurred the movement of the Savannah depot to Macon staring in late April 1862; the Charleston depot to Columbia, South Carolina, in May 1862; and the Atlanta depot to Augusta in July 1864. The Jackson depot was burned in May 1863 by Federal troops; its director, Surgeon Potts, had moved portions of his supplies to Mobile and dispersed some to other depots. Some depot purveyors included their purveying district number when identifying themselves, perhaps as a way of emphasizing their differentiation from field purveyors or from military commands. Newspaper advertisements, for example, showed Surgeon Prioleau representing the "4th Depot" (southern Georgia) and Surgeon George S. Blackie representing the "5th Depot" (northern Georgia).[17]

Field purveyors were to keep enough supplies for a month, but this could be a large amount of material since they were responsible for replenishing stores for an army or corps. Thus, they established their own depots, which could be more or less permanent, depending on the movement of their military command. Assistant Surgeon Zachary B. Herndon, medical purveyor for the Army of Northern Virginia, for example, received orders from General Lee in October 1862 to move his stores from Winchester to Staunton, Virginia, to establish a depot from which to supply the army. The longstanding depots in Wytheville and Mobile may have been established by field purveyors as well.[18]

In late 1864 and early 1865, district depots still existed in Richmond, Charlotte, Columbia (originally Charleston), Macon (originally Savannah), Augusta (originally Atlanta), and Montgomery. In addition to the officers in charge of those facilities, twenty-six additional purveyors appeared on a November 1864 list supplied by the SGO. Most appear to have been field purveyors, but actual positions are difficult to determine for the eight serving west of the Mississippi River in Arkansas, Louisiana, Texas, and the District of Indian Territory. Medical Department operations there came under primary control of the commander of the Trans-Mississippi Department after Union forces gained control of the river with the capture of Vicksburg in July 1863. Communication across the Mississippi became unreliable, and informative records of Trans-Mississippi medical purveying operations during the second half of the war are scarce.[19]

The Medical Laboratories

The medicines needed by the Confederate army were enumerated in a standard supply table adapted from US Army medical regulations. Before the war, the South had obtained those medicines for civilian use primarily from Northern merchants, who either imported the items or produced them in their own manufactories. Since the war curtailed trade with the North and engendered a naval blockade, Surgeon General Moore created establishments to manufacture standard army medicines and process indigenous plants for medicinal use.[20]

Perhaps the earliest evidence of such a facility is the request from Medical Purveyor Johns on January 22, 1862, to have Private Charles P. Sengstack of the First Virginia Infantry detailed to the "Medical Laboratory of the Purveyor's Department" in Richmond. After he had left the laboratory, Sengstack described himself as a "Practical Druggist of the Philadelphia school" who loved the "art of the manufacturing branch" but disapproved of "the manner in which Surgeon Johns treated his subordinates." Other laboratories arose in Alabama (Mobile and Montgomery), Arkansas (Little Rock and Arkadelphia, the latter relocated to Tyler, Texas), Georgia (Macon and Atlanta, the latter relocated to Augusta), Mississippi (Jackson), North Carolina (Charlotte and Lincolnton), and South Carolina (Columbia).[21]

With a few exceptions, medical laboratories were connected with and under the direction of depot purveyors. Facilities that encompassed both depots and laboratories could be quite large. In late 1864, for example, the Richmond depot-laboratory complex employed ninety men, exclusive of officers, and at one time included ten women in its workforce. The Arkansas and Texas facilities appear to have been operated by medical officers (surgeons in charge) who interacted closely with medical purveyors but did not hold that title themselves; those laboratories may also have served the Ordnance Department. The Lincolnton facility, operated by Surgeon in Charge Aaron Snowden Piggot, was the only medical laboratory east of the Mississippi River not directed by a medical purveyor and not an appendage of a purveying depot. When a purveyor's assistance was needed, Piggot turned to Surgeon James T. Johnson, the purveyor at Charlotte, about thirty miles away. In November 1864 his workforce, exclusive of officers, included forty men; whether he employed women is unknown. Some depots were associated with Confederate-operated distilleries for the manufacture of medicinal whiskey (see chapter 7).[22]

The number of employees at the medical-purveying depots, laboratories, and distilleries who were able-bodied yet designated as indispensable in late 1864 drew a protest from General Lee, who needed men to bolster his army.[23] In February 1865 Moore made his case to Secretary of War John C. Breckinridge:

> The employés of the laboratories, purveying depots, and distilleries are in a great measure expert chemists, druggists, and distillers, and men of professional skill, whose services are absolutely indispensable. . . . It is therefore hoped that the Honorable Secretary will see the necessity of these men being permanently attached to the Medical Department, as the practice of constantly changing these employés is productive of delay and embarrassment to the department. It is also important that they should be exempt from all military duty, for if called out in an emergency, when the purveyor is called upon to fill requisitions for the wounded, it is evident that suffering must ensue in consequence of their absence. Medical supplies can only be put up by skilled druggists.[24]

Later that month Moore mentioned the establishment of seven laboratories—in Lincolnton, Charlotte, Columbia, Macon, Atlanta, Mobile, and Montgomery—but his listing was inaccurate in terms of original or surviving facilities. The Atlanta laboratory, for example, had by then moved to Augusta, and Moore had ordered the Mobile laboratory closed in February 1863. Another late-war report, from October 1864, showed laboratories in Lincolnton,

Columbia, Macon, Augusta, and Tyler. By 1875 Moore had evidently forgotten the magnitude of laboratory operations when he recalled there being only three facilities east and one facility west of the Mississippi River.[25]

Surgeon General Moore—probably with assistance from Surgeon Johns—established a robust network of medical purveyors, purveying depots, and laboratories to furnish surgeons with medicines and other supplies. That network, in which Moore took a particular interest, turned to sources both foreign and domestic in an attempt to meet the needs of medical officers in the field and in hospitals.

6. ❖ Importation of Medical Supplies

Many of the supplies purchased by the Medical Department, including drugs, were imported, and having an adequate stock of medicines was mentioned after the war by both Jefferson Davis and Samuel Preston Moore as being of particular concern. To understand the problems faced by the Confederates in obtaining medicines, it is useful to examine the prewar drug market as it related to the items that the Southern military would desire. Medical supplies deemed appropriate for American troops were set forth in the US Army Medical Department's standard supply table, the last prewar version of which was issued in August 1860. Those used by the Confederate Medical Department throughout the war almost exactly reproduced that table. Each reflected the therapeutic philosophy of orthodox (regular or allopathic) physicians rather than that of one or more of the various medical sects (such as eclectic, reform, Thomsonian, and homeopathic) that were active at the time.[1]

A large proportion of the table's medicines were of vegetable origin. Some of the relevant plants grew in North America, but a great proportion did not, so many different roots, barks, seeds, leaves, and so on had to be imported. Many other medicinal substances, sometimes called chemicals (for example, chloroform and acids), were also imported to a large extent, especially if their constituent parts were abundant overseas. Before the war, some two-thirds to three-quarters of foreign medical goods into the United States arrived at New York City, with most of the rest shipped to Boston, Philadelphia, or Baltimore. Importers in those cities supplied wholesale druggists in interior parts of the country, retail druggists, and physicians. Wholesale druggists from the interior and local druggists typically traveled to one of the large importing centers periodically, visited a number of suppliers to personally examine their wares, and purchased a large stock of items without necessarily limiting themselves to one particular vendor. Customers who found such travel inconvenient typically formed a relationship with one wholesaler, with whom they placed orders for their medicinal stock by mail on six- or twelve-month credit.[2]

Some medicinal items available from importers or wholesalers—quinine sulfate, for example—were ready for an apothecary's shelves. Quinine, which was commonly used for malaria, was produced by manufacturing chemists in England, France, and Germany from the bark of South American cinchona trees and shipped to the United States, where an apothecary could incorporate it into prescriptions. Alternatively, manufacturing chemists could purchase cinchona bark from an importer or wholesaler and endeavor to produce their own quinine. The process was relatively complex, and at the time of the Civil War, only two American firms, both in the North, manufactured the drug. Depending on their expertise and time commitments, individual apothecaries could prepare other medicines from raw materials themselves or purchase them from manufacturing chemists.[3]

Despite the fact that many prewar Southern drug wholesalers called themselves importers, almost all of the foreign articles that they carried had originally been shipped into Northern ports, primarily New York, and then transported South. In the year ending June 30, 1859, for example, the value of opium imported into New York was $215,983; the corresponding value for New Orleans, the only Southern port receiving that drug, was $97. Southern wholesalers and apothecaries bought almost all of their stock from Northern wholesalers; transactions between New York wholesalers and Southern customers were brisk in 1859 and much of 1860. The secession crisis, however, prompted many Northern drug sellers to decline Southern orders for fear that payments would not be made. A Confederate tariff taking effect in March 1861 imposed a duty on goods entering the South from the North, so large orders were placed and filled to beat the deadline. Many Southern apothecaries stopped ordering from the North because they feared not being able to pay or thought that their orders would never arrive once hostilities began.[4]

After war broke out, regular drug business between Northern wholesalers and Southern customers stopped. In April 1861 President Lincoln first proclaimed a blockade of the ports of seven seceded states and then extended the blockade to include the ports of two other Southern states. He also issued a proclamation on August 16 prohibiting commercial dealings (unless exceptions were granted) between the North and the states in insurrection. Drugs were among the articles considered contraband of war by Secretary of the Treasury Salmon P. Chase. The Confederacy never barred importation of Northern goods during the war.[5]

Surgical instruments were also considered contraband of war. There were few instrument makers in the South, and most such items used by Southern surgeons were made in the North or in Europe. The vast majority of Confederate medical officers had been civilians immediately before the war. Many had not routinely performed major surgical procedure and thus did not own a set of instruments useful for military use. Those who did might well prefer to work with government-supplied sets rather than risk loss or damage of their own.[6]

The state of affairs might not be profoundly problematic if hostilities between North and South were short lived. Some Southern apothecaries had amassed an ample inventory of drugs and other medical supplies, and shortfalls might be supplemented by importations, especially if the US Navy could not immediately implement an effective blockade. Yet a prolonged conflict and an efficient blockade, combined with a large military force requiring care, would severely challenge the ability of medical officers of the Confederate army to obtain adequate supplies of medical goods.

Purchases in Europe

Confederate officials recognized early the need to increase imports into their ports and sent agents to Europe to buy supplies and send them across the Atlantic. Shipment was initially in large steamers that went directly to the South, but such ships were vulnerable to Union blockaders. There then evolved the practice of large vessels laden with European goods stopping at the neutral ports of Nassau (in the Bahamas) or Bermuda. Cargos would be unloaded there in exchange for cotton, which was carried back to Europe. Goods unloaded at Nassau or Bermuda were placed, at the direction of Confederate agents, on swift, shallow-draft steamers that could more easily elude blockaders and slip into Southern ports such as Wilmington, Charleston, or Savannah. Crews then traded their cargo for cotton, which they carried back to Nassau or Bermuda to be placed on the larger vessels and transported to Europe. Shipping routes could also consist of a stop at Cuba and final transshipment to Matamoros, Mexico, where the unloaded goods would be transported overland into the Confederate Trans-Mississippi District. Space in vessels not taken by supplies already purchased by the Confederate government was used to carry goods, including medical supplies, predicted by their owners to bring a good price at auction, whether the buyer was the government or another customer.[7]

It appears that artillery captain (later major) Caleb Huse was the first man dispatched to Europe whose duties included the procurement of medical supplies for the Confederacy. Huse was ordered on April 15, 1861, to act as the government's agent "for the purchase of ordnance, arms, equipments, and military stores." Details of his mission would come from Colonel Josiah Gorgas, chief of ordnance, but Huse was also to follow instructions from "heads of other departments of this Government in reference to their several departments." His efforts resulted in huge amounts of supplies—mostly for the Ordnance Department—being shipped to the Confederacy. After the quartermaster general complained about the officer's fitness to purchase for that department, Huse was directed to purchase for the Ordnance and Medical Departments only. According to Gorgas, Surgeon General Moore had full confidence in Huse's judgment.[8]

How much the surgeon general relied on Huse and what items he wished him to purchase are unknown, but communications to him from Moore provide a glimpse of their working relationship as it existed in mid-1863. The Medical Department appears to have decided during June 1863 to buy cotton and use it to pay for medical supplies in Europe. To avoid competition among the various branches of the Confederate government in these purchases, Moore obtained approval from the secretary of the treasury to make them through approved agents. He then ordered Medical Purveyor George S. Blackie in Atlanta to place an order for 2,000 bales and pay for it with $500,000 made available to him for hospital supplies. Blackie was to have the cotton delivered to James M. Seixas, agent at Charleston, who would arrange for its shipment to Europe. Moore informed Huse that arrangements had been made to purchase 6,250 bales of cotton for shipment to England—Blackie was evidently not the only purveyor involved—where credit for its sale could be used by Huse to buy items for the Medical Department. The surgeon general provided him a list of supplies to purchase and ship to the Confederacy. In another communication, this in October 1863, Moore informed him that the Medical Department had on hand cotton worth $1.5 million, that medical purveyors were buying more projected to be worth an additional £1 million, and that the funds would be available to him for future purchases. Huse was to ship the purchased supplies "in divided lots, so that each shipment shall consist of a *portion* of each article of supply, so that, in the event of capture or loss by sea, the whole of any one article may not be lost." Because Southern cotton purchased by the Medical Department was transported by Ordnance Department steamers to the intermediate points of Bermuda or Nassau, Moore asked Huse to apply a credit to that department for every pound of Medical Department cotton arriving in England as payment for transportation charges.[9]

Among other individuals attempting to buy supplies abroad were A. F. D. Gifford and Nathaniel Beverly Tucker, who asked President Davis on July 17, 1861, to authorize their travel to Europe to obtain military stores. The men suggested that they could "purchase any thing and every thing which the army required, and which, for the present, could not be purchased in this Country." Possibly because of turnover in the War Department—Leroy P. Walker was replaced by Judah P. Benjamin in September 1861—communication about the proposal suffered, but on October 1 Quartermaster General Abraham C. Myers suggested to Benjamin that the pair be authorized to "deliver the articles in one of our ports at their risk." According to Tucker, he and Gifford were "intrusted by the Ordnance, Quartermaster's, and Surgeon-General's Departments . . . with orders to a large amount to be purchased in Europe and shipped to the Confederate States." The surgeon general's involvement in this assignment is unknown.[10]

Gifford left Savannah on the steamer *Bermuda* in early November 1861 and made purchases in Europe. In the meantime Tucker endured delays in transportation and finally arrived in England in February 1862, long after Gifford had departed London (December 24, 1861) on a return voyage "in a steamer fitted out with a valuable cargo for the Confederate States." The cargo was said to include "articles greatly needed in the Confederacy, such as medicines, &c, &c." The vessel was never heard from, presumed to be lost at sea, and Tucker was left without his friend Gifford and the money he had raised for the expedition. It appears that he did not try again to purchase medical supplies for the benefit of the Confederacy, although he went to Canada in 1864 to help procure food for the army. Tucker was also accused, evidently wrongly, with complicity in the assassination of President Lincoln.[11]

Augustus Coutanche Evans was yet another agent dispatched to Europe. A native North Carolinian, Evans had graduated with a medical degree from the University of Pennsylvania and worked as a wholesale druggist in New York City. He returned south shortly after the war began and approached Secretary of War Walker on July 2, 1861, in hopes of traveling to Europe to purchase medical supplies for the Confederacy. On being asked to prepare a written proposal, Evans then visited Acting Surgeon General David Camden DeLeon to ascertain exactly what supplies were needed. DeLeon was unable to respond immediately but later sent him "a list of such articles as form an outfit in his department, but without specifying such as would be required." Moore, after replacing DeLeon as acting surgeon general, again informed

Evans what was desired, and the agent departed for Europe "to make purchase of certain drugs and medical supplies."[12]

Evans sailed from Savannah in late 1861 on the *Bermuda*, the same vessel carrying the ill-fated A. F. D. Gifford, but evidently had little financial support from the Confederate government. Despite a request from Surgeon General Moore that the agent receive £20,000 from Huse for purchases, Evans was unable to fill Moore's order. He did report that he "lost no opportunity in persuading shipments of medicines and was instrumental in having shipped a large amt, some considerable quantity of which was captured." Evans returned from Europe in late September 1862 and offered again to help the government, either by providing advice or returning to Europe to try purchasing again. Although he was apparently in poor health on his return to North Carolina, he was appointed as assistant surgeon of a North Carolina regiment; he died in February 1863.[13]

Role of Neutral Ports

Bermuda was a key intermediate point in the acquisition of supplies from Europe. Confederate representatives there bought and shipped goods at the request of Surgeon General Moore. In August 1863, for example, Major Smith Stansbury, a Confederate officer commanding the ordnance depot in Bermuda, informed Moore that he had purchased brandy on his order and would arrange shipping to Wilmington as quickly as he could. During the same month, Stansbury informed Major Norman S. Walker—another ordnance officer who was a disbursing agent in Bermuda—that he would bid for brandy to help fill an order from the Medical Department. Stansbury was clearly dealing with goods that had not already been purchased by Confederate agents in Europe.[14]

Nassau handled a larger proportion than Bermuda of goods bound for Southern ports. While a large percentage of such items arrived directly at Nassau from Europe (primarily England), a portion arrived from ports in the United States. The British consul in Charleston, Robert Bunch, described in April 1862 how such transactions occurred: "The Richmond Government sent about a month ago an order to Nassau for Medicines, Quinine, etc. It went from Nassau to New York, was executed there, came back to Nassau, thence here, and was on its way to Richmond in 21 days from the date of the order. Nearly all the trade is under British flag." Hiram Barney, with the New York Custom House, reported that companies known to be hostile to the United States had warehouses in the city that served as "the depot for goods awaiting shipment to rebel ports on the order and under the direction of rebel agents resident at Nassau." This mode of shipment developed, in part, because of the danger of the US Navy's blockading force capturing cargoes from Europe bound for Nassau or Bermuda and because of quarantines imposed in response to outbreaks of yellow fever at those ports. Thus, British shippers at times sent their goods first to New York for later transport, in vessels flying the British flag, to Nassau under the assumption that the United States would not interfere with shipments from its own ports to neutral ports. Shipment of war materiel from Northern ports to Nassau often—perhaps usually—contained goods of US origin. A witness testifying before a US House committee stated, "I have seen large quantities of goods landed at Nassau (such as boots and shoes, cloth and clothing, provisions, drugs and medicines, blankets marked U.S.A., liquors, &c.,) from vessels arriving from New York, Boston, and Baltimore, and have afterwards seen portions of the same goods being shipped on board blockade-runners for Wilmington and other rebel ports." The British government argued that US officials should allow "articles of innocent use" to be shipped from Northern ports to Nassau, but Barney contended that such articles, clearly intended for the Confederacy, had included "sulphate of quinine in quantities of one thousand ounces, chloroform by the hundred pounds, surgical instruments by the dozen cases," and other valuable supplies.[15]

Materials lying in storage at neutral ports and not already purchased by or reserved for the Confederate government could be bought through representatives of importing companies. An agent for the owners of the steamer *Theodora*, for example, soon to depart Charleston for Havana, informed Medical Purveyor Chisolm that the vessel could return with medicines. Chisolm asked Surgeon General Moore on November 30, 1861, for a list of desired items, but a reply arrived shortly after the steamer had sailed on December 4 (for Nassau rather than Cuba). Moore was given another chance to place an order in late December for another trip by the same vessel, which by that time had been purchased by the Confederate government and renamed *Nassau*. Chisolm noted in September 1862 that prices in Nassau were much lower than in Charleston and thus justified running the risk that goods purchased in the Bahamas might be lost during transit to the Southern states. He thus asked Surgeon Edward W. Johns, medical purveyor in Richmond, for permission to place orders. It was evidently granted, for Chisolm placed his own orders with importing companies in Nassau and asked Confederate agents there to assist in shipping the goods to Charleston. Johns's Circular Nos. 1 and 3, issued in April 1862, directed depot purveyors at marine ports of entry, such as Chisolm, to immediately take advantage of "opportunities to import supplies" if waiting for Johns's approval might result in loss of those chances. It is unclear if Johns was encouraging purveyors to initiate importation or was simply referring to purchasing already landed imports, but Chisolm took the safe route and sought permission to place orders.[16]

Buying Imports in the Southern Market

During the time that Johns had some supervisory authority over medical purveyors—April 7, 1862, to February 25, 1863—he issued many orders regarding the imported medical goods that had reached the South. Available records do not indicate the extent to which his actions simply reflected the desires of the surgeon general, but Johns referred various matters to Moore, who issued his own instructions to purveyors during that time. It seems likely that Moore at least made overarching decisions during that span, such as those regarding impressment and pricing guidelines. Outside of that time span, decisions regarding imported goods can more confidently be attributed to the surgeon general or at least to his staff in the SGO.

Moore bypassed Johns on July 11, 1862, by ordering Medical Purveyor William H. Prioleau at Savannah to report on the number of surgical-operating cases he had on hand and how many consisted of high-quality instruments from England; he was to send one English set to Johns to be forwarded to the SGO. Prioleau reported that he had nine "very complete and valuable" English sets and was negotiating for the purchase of eighteen more that had recently arrived on the blockade-runner *Thomas L. Wragg*. Although the owner of the *Wragg*'s instruments wanted $400 each for the six finest cases and $200 each for the other twelve—twice what Prioleau was originally willing to pay—Johns ordered him to buy all eighteen sets, sending the best ones to Richmond and keeping the lower-priced ones to be issued from Savannah. Prioleau had earlier reported having "English cases for general operation far too good to be issued to the majority of surgeons in service around this place. They are just the thing for General Hospitals." Moore and Johns evidently agreed.[17]

Johns was kept informed of a problem stemming from an early agreement with a Southern importing company. In September or October 1861, Medical Director and Purveyor Alexander N. Talley contracted with John Ashhurst and Company of Charleston for the latter to import supplies sufficient for 100,000 men for a year; the material was to be delivered January–March

1862 at Charleston and paid for as it arrived. The shipments were late, and disagreements arose between Ashhurst and Assistant Surgeon Prioleau (by then medical purveyor at Savannah) about prices for goods. The supplies in question were aboard the steamer *Kate*, which docked at Savannah on June 30; its intended port seems to have been Charleston. By that time the contract had expired, and Ashhurst evidently claimed, to Prioleau's surprise, that *Kate*'s medical supplies were not part of the government order.[18] When Prioleau informed Surgeon Johns of this, the latter advised:

> Several parties have contracted with the Government for large quantities of medical supplies to be delivered about this time in Confederate ports, and it is not improbable that some of the cargoes recently arriving may be diverted from their legitimate direction and advantage taken of the present inflated condition of the market and offered for sale to others. In view of this probability you are instructed to make diligent enquiry in every instance and if such advantage should be sought, you will, through the agency of the Provost Marshall, resort to impressment under the authority vested in me by the Secretary of War a copy of which I enclose herewith. In other cases you will purchase at reasonable prices if practicable otherwise impress for use of Government, and a fair valuation can be subsequently determined.[19]

The permission mentioned by Johns came from Secretary of War Randolph on June 18: "Impressment may be made whenever necessary for the Army but the operations of trade should be interfered with as little as possible. Care must be taken not to interrupt the supplies necessary and such interruptions must be solely to supply the Army and not with the view of controlling trade."[20]

Prioleau had *Kate*'s medical cargo seized. Although Ashhurst professed a patriotic desire to sell to the government at reduced but fair prices, he deemed those offered to him by Prioleau unsatisfactory. The discussion eventually turned heated, and Ashhurst resolved to "refer the matter to the Surgeon General at Richmond, who will doubtless take a business view of the case, and abide his decision in the premises." The outcome of the dispute is known, but Prioleau, who feared that Moore would disapprove of his actions, remained in his position for the rest of the war.[21]

The *Kate* incident, in fact, was not the first time that the Medical Department considered impressment. In late May 1862 Johns ordered Chisolm to impress goods that he had ordered from Duncan, Williams, and Company of New Orleans and was expected "at some convenient Confederate Port." (It is unclear whether the company had the goods in stock or was acting as an agent in importing them from Nassau, Bermuda, or Cuba.) Chisolm consequently ordered one of his agents, Charles Edmondston, to make offers for all medical stores recently imported into Charleston. He authorized the agent to pay prices he had recently allowed, which still provided wholesalers handsome profits. If merchants demanded exorbitant prices, Edmondston was to "quietly seize" the supplies with the help of the local military commander.[22]

On May 31, Johns instructed Chisolm and Prioleau to "press all the medicines in the principal cities in your district to make up a supply for 200,000 men for six months, leaving in the apothecaries' hands only such supplies as are necessary to meet their prescription business." He allowed for liberal but not exorbitant prices. Chisolm and Prioleau were to act simultaneously so that merchants would not have time to remove their goods to avoid seizure. The aggressive procurement of materials was spurred, in part, by looming military action. On May 27, for example, Chisolm instructed his agent to ship chloroform to Richmond "to be at hand for the great Battle now hourly expected" (probably the Battle of Seven Pines, May 31–June 1, 1862). In response to orders to impress all medical goods, in September 1862 he suggested to Johns that items not currently needed by the Medical Department be left alone so that they would be available for public sale and thus help keep overall prices down.[23]

Fabrics were among the seized goods after the steamer *Cuba* arrived at St. Marks, Florida, in January 1863. These were transported by railroad at government expense to Houston, Florida, where they were received by Surgeon J. E. A. Davidson, the medical purveyor stationed at Quincy, before being turned over to Medical Purveyor George S. Blackie at Atlanta. In February 1863, just before Johns was relieved of his supervisory duties over other purveyors, the surgeon general instructed Blackie on disbursing *Cuba*'s cloth and other goods: "The Calico is probably not too inferior for comforts, the canvas is needed for field stretchers, and the kerosene oil is intended for lanterns in field service." Prices to be paid for the cargo were determined by a board of survey but were too low to satisfy the vessel's owners.[24]

Medical purveyors also obtained imported goods through public auctions organized by companies associated with blockade-runners. Purveyors were careful not to bid against each other, while cautioning their agents at such auctions to conceal their association with the Medical Department.[25]

Trading with the Enemy

As previously mentioned, some supplies bound for the Southern states arrived at neutral ports from Northern shipping centers, sent by merchants who had no qualms about their supplies ending up in Confederate hands as long as the profits were good. There was also a thriving market in Union-controlled areas within the Southern states. There, currency and medical and other vital supplies from the North were traded for cotton.

Union and Confederate policies and practices regarding trading with the enemy were inconsistent and confusing (and will not be discussed here). Suffice it to say that such commerce was common and practiced by Confederate officials desperate for vital supplies. One Federal officer described Union-occupied Memphis, for example, as more valuable than Nassau to the Confederacy: "The practical operation of commercial intercourse from this city with the States in rebellion has been to help largely to feed, clothe, arm and equip our enemies. . . . To take cotton belonging to the Government to Nassau, or any foreign port, is a hazardous proceeding. To take it to Memphis and convert it to supplies and greenbacks and return to the lines of the enemy, or place the proceeds to the credit of the rebel Government in Europe, without passing again into rebel lines, is safe and easy."[26]

Surgeon Edward N. Covey was a medical inspector in October 1864 and recognized how effective the blockade was becoming. In one inspection report he urged Surgeon General Moore to take advantage of the opportunity to trade cotton for Northern medical supplies:

> If the business were entrusted to an active and enterprising Purveyor, I am fully satisfied that a large amount of supplies could be purchased from the enemy's lines at various points along the Mississippi river at much reduced prices compared to those now paid in the open market. . . . This trade was carried on at one time by the Government for the benefit of the Ordnance Department, and small lots of medicines have in the same way been purchased for our Department by the agents controlling the business—as matters of favors—but no active or well arranged efforts have ever been made to carry on the trade by our Department. . . . Surgeon [Richard] Potts, from his position, his excellent business qualifications and his knowledge of the men in business, both within our lines and in our cities within the lines of the enemy, I consider the

best man to entrust with this business. . . . As the port of Mobile, and in fact all the ports as high up as Wilmington No. Ca. are probably closed during the War, and all ingress of supplies stopped, and as transportation from N.C. is expensive, difficult and uncertain, I would respectfully recommend that Surg. Potts be entrusted with the experiment with the belief that it will prove a success. Only one thing is necessary to its perfect success and that is, that he shall control at all times the cotton and be able to direct its shipment to points of delivery of medicines.

In a personal note to Potts, Covey urged, "By all means get control of the cotton and its shipment or the whole thing will be a fizzle."[27]

Potts had in fact been authorized by the surgeon general no later than December 1862 to acquire supplies over enemy lines, but his activities had been impeded by Confederate officials who either disallowed agreements that he had made or refused to supply the cotton that he intended to use as payment. "There is nothing to prevent my getting as many supplies as I wish," wrote Potts to Moore in August 1864, "if I only have the thing fixed so that I cannot be interfered with." Potts, who was operating in southern Mississippi and eastern Louisiana, asked the surgeon general to get an order from the secretary of the treasury for a large amount of cotton to be turned over to him in his region and an order from the secretary of war allowing him to transport the cotton through the lines to pay for the goods. In September 1864 he became aware that Medical Purveyor Robinson Miller at Mobile was arranging similar goods-for-cotton deals. Potts asked him to annul his contracts because having another purveyor vying for supplies would drive up their cost. "I have been placed in charge of all that business by the Surgeon General," he informed Miller. In light of Potts's long history of trading through the lines, Surgeon Covey's aforementioned communication to the surgeon general was not merely a suggestion that Potts become involved in trade but rather an appeal that he be given full control of such dealings.[28]

Moore replied on February 9, 1865, that Potts had been given "exclusive control of the importation of such articles as are most needed, until recent orders from the War Department, taking entire control of transactions of this nature, [had] impaired his usefulness and put a stop in a measure to the supply." He projected that trade through the lines on the Mississippi River and along the Gulf border of Mississippi and Alabama would be the Medical

Department's chief source of supply "in consequence of the recent disaster at Wilmington." Moore was referring to the fall of Fort Fisher the previous month, which would enable Union forces to capture Wilmington, the Confederacy's busiest port for blockade-runners, the last of which to arrive being the *Wild Rover* on December 28, 1864. He urged the secretary of war to allow Potts to resume his trading activities. How effective the surgeon general's appeal was is unclear, but it came too late to have much effect on the war.[29]

Missions to the North

Smuggling from the North by civilians, on their own, and the capture of Union supplies by Confederate forces occasionally provided the Medical Department with much-needed material. Such episodes, however, were outside of the surgeon general's control and are not discussed here. In one case, after a Mr. Block proposed crossing enemy lines to procure medical goods, the secretary of war expressed a willingness to grant permission for the surgeon general to contract with the man or with "any agency he [the surgeon general] may appoint" to secure the supplies.[30]

In some instances the Medical Department directed military personnel to procure goods from the North. For example, in July 1863, immediately after the Battle of Gettysburg, Moore ordered Surgeon Covey and Assistant Surgeons Thomas S. Latimer and Ignatius D. Thomson to proceed into Maryland to purchase and collect medical supplies in the rear of Lee's army in that state and in Pennsylvania. The outcome of that mission remains unknown.[31]

A few months later, in October 1863, the secretary of war issued permits to J. J. Crawford, Asa H. Balderston, and Joseph A. Fedderman to pass Confederate lines into the United States and return with supplies for the Medical Department as specified by Medical Purveyor Johns. The permits prohibited the men from engaging in "any private adventure" and confined each to "act strictly as an agent for the Department that confides business to his charge, as this Department cannot license any individual enterprise of trade with the enemy." Crawford's identity is uncertain, but he may have been James J. Crawford, an experienced druggist who was appointed as a hospital steward in September 1864. Balderston, a dentist, had worked at the medical-purveying depot in Richmond and then as a volunteer or contract surgeon at the Blind Asylum Hospital in Macon; he became a Confederate hospital steward in 1865 and performed dental services. At about the time of his assignment,

Fedderman was being discharged as a private from the Thirty-Ninth Virginia Infantry. The overall success of the men is unknown, but Fedderman's mission did not end well.[32]

By late January 1864 Fedderman was confined at the Old Capital Prison in Washington, DC. By late July he was on his way to Albany (New York) Penitentiary after a US military commission convicted him—evidently as a US citizen rather than as a Confederate agent or spy—of "trading with the enemy." According to a Washington newspaper, Fedderman purchased contraband goods in Baltimore and elsewhere in the United States; turned them over to the enemy in Northumberland County, Virginia; and returned to the United States without authority. His prison sentence was to last "until the termination of the present rebellion." In response to an appeal from Fedderman's father, which was supported by a Union general and others, President Lincoln ordered the younger Fedderman's release from prison on March 9, 1865, "to remain at liberty so long as he does not hereafter misbehave."[33]

The tactic of sending men to the North was likely to yield relatively small amounts of supplies. That it was undertaken suggests the tenuous nature of the Medical Department's supply situation and the lack of confidence that other means would deliver goods in adequate quantities.

Obtaining goods from foreign countries, including the United States, was a key strategy for maintaining adequate stores of medical supplies. It was never sufficient, however, and could not be sustained even at that level if the Union naval blockade became more effective. Thus, Surgeon General Moore also directed medical purveyors to purchase from domestic suppliers, harvest and process indigenous medicinal resources, and establish facilities to manufacture medicines.

7. ❧ Turning to Domestic Resources

Although Confederate officials devoted considerable attention to importing medical supplies, there were sources of medical goods within the Southern states themselves. Thus, as described in chapter 1, materials at US military facilities in the South were seized even before hostilities began with Fort Sumter. The eagerness of Southern civilians to assist the army prompted the Provisional Congress to pass a bill, approved in August 1861, directing the appointment of a special clerk in the SGO to take charge of all supplies donated for the sick and wounded. H. T. Banks was subsequently appointed contribution clerk and placed under the orders of Surgeon Edward W. Johns, medical purveyor for Richmond. The Medical Department also took advantage of the South's material and human resources by buying supplies already in the hands of merchants, entering into contracts with individuals or firms to collect or produce needed goods, and establishing or taking control of manufacturing facilities. Over time, the department generally moved away from contracts and toward arrangements with greater government control.[1]

Purchasing or Impressing Existing Stock

Early in the war, medical purveyors could take advantage of merchants' relatively plentiful inventories. When Assistant Surgeon William H. Prioleau assumed responsibility as medical purveyor at Savannah in March 1862, medical purveyor Surgeon J. J. Chisolm at Charleston, to whom Prioleau was initially subordinate, instructed him to purchase from a large and reliable drug supplier. "They may do most of the business for you," advised Chisolm, "and to a great extent may render a large [medical purveying] establishment unnecessary." Some of the goods owned by apothecaries may have been stockpiled before hostilities began, but much of what they provided had recently arrived through the blockade. In any event, the mode of business suggested by Chisolm removed the need to deal with overseas agents or to bid at auctions for the cargoes of blockade-runners. Prioleau had another reason to heed this advice: The recent fall of Fort Pulaski, at the mouth of the Savannah River, meant that Savannah was under the threat of capture. In late April 1862 Prioleau informed Medical Purveyor Johns in Richmond that, "owing to this City being threatened, I have refrained from purchasing a large supply of Drugs, preferring to keep what I have in safety and making use of the city Druggists to fill my requisitions, which should the City be taken will save a great many Drugs to the Confederacy, as those owned by Government will be saved and the Stocks of the Druggists will have been reduced in the service of the Government."[2]

A. A. Solomons and Company, a Savannah-based operation, was Prioleau's principal supplier at the time and shared his anxiety. According to the assistant surgeon, "They have a large stock on hand, too large they say for them to risk, but if the Government will indemnify them for a portion should the City be taken, they will risk it. Otherwise they will send it away, which would put me to a great deal of inconvenience unless I keep a large stock myself." Johns consulted the surgeon general about the danger to Savannah and relayed a decision: "The Government will take no risk and you are instructed to purchase supplies necessary and move them to Macon. Purchase to good advantage *not stating* that you will remove the articles bought to Macon. If the prices asked are too high you will be furnished with supplies from Charleston from supplies arriving from Europe."[3]

Prioleau moved much of his inventory to Macon and ended up, with other medical purveyors, buying supplies in large amounts and storing them in depots per Johns's Circular No. 3 (April 1862). The only large port in Prioleau's purveying district, Savannah, was not a particularly active one for blockade-runners, so he was forced to purchase goods that had entered through other ports. Those supplies might be offered at auctions held at various sites in his district or purchased from merchants who had obtained the items from blockade-runners for their own inventory or to resell; prices in the South were rising quickly, and speculation could be quite profitable. Prioleau's situation was shared by other depot purveyors not as fortunate as Chisolm, who had the active blockade-running ports of Charleston and Wilmington in his district.[4]

Impressment, which was employed selectively and with approval from Richmond, could be used not only to gain possession of imported items thought to have been ordered by the Medical Department but also to secure favorable prices for goods already in the hands of local merchants. Medical Purveyor Chisolm, for example, offered to obtain supplies at Charleston for fellow medical purveyor George S. Blackie at Atlanta by using his "privilege of impressment." According to Chisolm, prices paid for impressed goods were at least 50 percent lower than those that he would have to pay otherwise. He thought this "privilege" was an important tactic for combatting speculation, a belief shared by other purveying personnel. "I have telegraphed you to get a general order to impress quinine," wrote James Stewart, a purveying assistant, to Prioleau during Stewart's purchasing travels throughout Georgia. "I have found traces of some one to three hundred ounces in the hands of speculators in Columbus." Blackie told Prioleau that he was seeking permission to seize quinine from speculators in his district. "I trust I may get it," he said, "and disappoint the greedy bloodsuckers who are so abundant at this time." Purveyors were mindful not to be too aggressive with impressment. When Prioleau and Chisolm coordinated with each other in impressing goods, they took care to leave adequate supplies in the hands of apothecaries so that they could continue their regular prescription business.[5]

Supplies Other Than Medicines

Purveyors used special strategies for obtaining surgical instruments already in Southern hands. They appealed to retired physicians and others to donate or sell their instruments to the Medical Department. Medical Purveyor Prioleau suggested that medical officers be permitted to sell their personal instruments to the government, continue to use them while in the army, and buy them back at the same price when they left the service. The government would thus assume the risk of the instruments being lost or damaged, and an incoming military surgeon would be less likely to leave his personal instruments safely at home. Under this arrangement, if instruments were lost or damaged through no fault of the surgeon, the price he needed to pay to regain ownership would be lowered. E. W. Johns approved Prioleau's plan, provided that appropriate records were kept, but then instructed him in August 1862 to discontinue this mode of procuring instruments.[6]

The South had few experienced makers of medical supplies, so the medical purveyor in Charleston was ordering the manufacture of tourniquets by June 1861 from saddle and harness maker A. McKensie and Company, cots by November 1861 from furniture dealer Benjamin and Goodrich (Augusta), and ball forceps by June 1862 from blacksmith F. W. Thauss. He also ordered medical knapsacks from an unidentified contractor. In Macon Prioleau bought field tourniquets and probangs (instruments for removing foreign bodies from the esophagus and trachea) made by Peter Straus and cupping tins made by Oliver and Douglass. Other firms making surgical instruments for the Confederacy included Julius Holtzscheiter of Tarboro, North Carolina; Louis Froelich and Company of Kenansville, North Carolina; and Delarue and Hyer of Richmond. Exactly what these firms made and in what numbers is unknown. Surgeon Lafayette Guild, medical director of the Army of Northern Virginia, was not impressed with the Southern-made implements he saw. "Many medical officers are illy supplied with surgical implements," he reported to Surgeon General Moore in April 1863. "Some, indeed to whom instruments of Confederate manufacture were issued," he continued, "might as well be without any, for those they have are entirely useless." Guild asked to be supplied with imported instruments. Moore recalled after the war that "a not very successful effort was made to manufacture operating-knives."[7]

By April 1862 Medical Purveyor Johns in Richmond was ordering bedsteads from lumber dealers Payne and Jackson of Petersburg, Virginia. Prioleau in Georgia dealt with Samuel L. Gustin of Macon for fabrics, the manufacture of bedding—sometimes using fabric supplied by the medical purveyor—and hospital knapsacks; Grenville Wood of Macon for bunks and medicine chests; and T. B. Marshall and Brother of Savannah for fabrics, stretchers, and hospital clothing.[8]

Surgeon General Moore complained late in the war that, since contracts for hospital furniture, bedding, and like items often went unfilled, his department began to assume direct control of the production of such articles, which involved the detailing of artisans from the ranks. It is unclear whether the Medical Department purchased factories or conducted manufacturing in its preexisting facilities, but many purveying depots employed carpenters who may have constructed simple items such as litters and bunks. An 1864 inspection of Surgeon Prioleau's Macon depot revealed that "the supply of Instruments was small but of a tolerably good quality except the cupping tins and field tourniquets both of which were very indifferent the latter were exceedingly indifferently made and of poor material," the report continuing, "bedding and clothing were manufactured of an excellent article of cotton cloth but not very well made," bunk legs were "at too great an angle with the body, and consequently break easily," and folding bunks and hospital knapsacks were "not very good." Despite these shortcomings, Surgeon General Moore told Prioleau, "the report however is in the main very favorable and I am pleased to see that your officers and employees are faithful in the performance of their duties and endeavoring to promote the best interests of the service." He undoubtedly understood how severely limited his purveyors were in obtaining materials and detailing skilled men to work for contractors or at government facilities.[9]

Alcohol

Alcohol, usually in the form of whiskey or brandy, was an important medicinal agent, but its acquisition posed particular problems for medical purveyors. Although the 1860 census showed 299 distilleries in the Southern states, they produced less than 2 percent of the whiskey and less than 1 percent of the brandy distilled in the entire United States. Southern liquor production dropped early in the war after distilleries were dismantled for the copper in their apparatus, the metal being needed for other war-related purposes. Medical purveyors contracted with individual distillers, but Moore noted that they often practiced "gross fraud" by producing more than their contract specified and offering "so indifferent and spurious an article that the department was obliged to reject it." The distillers then sold the excess or rejected liquor for higher prices than those in the government contracts.[10]

By early 1863 Moore determined that the expedient course would be for the Medical Department to purchase or establish its own distilleries. Resistance from Governors Joseph E. Brown of Georgia and Zebulon B. Vance of North Carolina, who maintained that grain should be used to feed the army and the citizenry rather than to make liquor, was met with legislation allowing the surgeon general and commissary general to contract or establish distilleries for the production of liquors. Those facilities operated by the Medical Department—generally associated with purveying depots—were in Montgomery, Alabama; Lewisville, Arkansas; Macon, Georgia; Salisbury and Lincolnton, North Carolina; Columbia, South Carolina; and Tyler, Texas.[11]

Harvesting Indigenous Resources

The collection of native medicinal plants—and the establishment of medical laboratories to process them (see chapter 5)—marked one of Surgeon General Moore's most assertive and practical decisions regarding the acquisition of medical supplies. He noted after the war, "It had been my impression for a long time that many of the southern medical plants possessed valuable properties, and that their usefulness would soon be discovered in many diseases if administered with care and attention." Indeed, many medicines used by both military and civilian practitioners were based on plants, and many of those found in the South were already known to be medicinally useful, although often not as the first choice of most practitioners. Perhaps Moore did not appreciate what was already known about Southern medicinal flora or, not having prescribed those species himself, did not know how they measured up to first-line remedies. A hospital steward who had once worked in the SGO referred to native plants as "those indigenous remedies that sit like a nightmare upon the brain of the Surgeon General." Regardless of whether Moore was truly obsessed, he displayed a keen and constant interest in indigenous flora and issued orders about their collection, even while Johns was serving as a supervisory purveyor. He expressed his general view about indigenous remedies: "It is not desirable that the list of articles employed should be multiplied. It is more important that a moderate number of the more valuable, should be selected and these prepared for use promptly and properly."[12]

An early indicator of Moore's interest may have been a December 1861 inquiry from Medical Purveyor Johns to Surgeon Chisolm as to whether "French willow" could be purchased in New Orleans and, if so, at what price. (Since Johns was not known to have a particular interest in medicinal flora, he was probably relaying a question from Moore.) Exactly what plant he meant and whether it grew along the Gulf coast or was imported are unclear, for the name could have referred to various species. In any case, Chisolm learned that French willow was unavailable in New Orleans. The plant may have been the same one described in April 1862 by Medical Purveyor Prioleau to Johns: "I enclose a few pieces of bark of willow imported to this City [Savannah]. The owner represents that it is largely used in the West Indies as a substitute for Quinine [for malaria]. Messrs. A. Solomons & Co have it for sale." Willow bark was indeed useful in malaria, but willow was abundant in the South, so it is unlikely that Prioleau was ordered to buy the imported bark.[13]

The distribution of the March 1862 pamphlet *General Directions for Collecting and Drying Medicinal Substances of the Vegetable Kingdom* marked the beginning of Moore's concerted effort to put native flora to good use. In the April 1862 circular accompanying the publication, the surgeon general announced: "It is the policy of all nations at all times, especially such as at present exists in our Confederacy, to make every effort to develop its internal resources, and to diminish its tribute to foreigners by supplying its necessities from the productions of its own soil. This observation may be considered peculiarly applicable to the appropriation of our indigenous medicinal substances of the vegetable kingdom." He went on to encourage medical officers to collect the species in the pamphlet and to assist in determining the clinical value of those and other plants. Johns's Circular No. 3, which was also issued in April 1862 and undoubtedly reflected Moore's desires, instructed medical purveyors to collect indigenous plants and to issue medicines made from them when standard remedies were in short supply. During the next month, Moore ordered Surgeon Francis Peyre Porcher to enlarge the March 1862 pamphlet (see chapter 12).[14]

In September 1862, amid Johns's tenure as so-called chief purveyor, Moore began issuing additional orders to medical purveyors about collecting and processing medicinal plants. Some instructions specified exactly which ones deserved the most attention and those whose collection could cease. Johns had ordered purveyors to place notices in newspapers showing prices offered for various plants and to send him copies of those announcements. Moore reacted to Medical Purveyor Prioleau's notice by comparing his prices with those paid by another purveyor, Assistant Surgeon W. B. Robertson, at Wytheville, Virginia. "For the Cranesbill for which you are paying $1.00 pr lb. he gives but 20 cts," he noted. "This plant where it grows, generally grows abundantly, but as it requires some trouble to prepare the root, i.e. removing the old & decayed root, from the newer, 30 or 40 cts would probably be a fairer price. . . . Of course, the general rule for fixing the prices should be the intrinsic importance of the article itself, taken in connection with its abundance in the vicinity, and the trouble of preparing it." In contrast with Moore, who in this instance allowed for judgment, Johns was more prescriptive in indicating a maximum price that purveyors should pay. Prioleau complained to him: "I do not think prices of these articles can be safely fixed where they are not to be found. . . . I am ordered by my Government to pay in some instance less than half of what I agreed. In future I shall make no agreement in price, for I value the reputation of my Government and myself too highly to have the charge of fickleness put upon us." Moore later specified maximum prices that Prioleau was to pay; if the purveyor objected, he apparently kept silent about it.[15]

In an unusual instance of animal material being sought, Moore directed purveyors to take steps to have potato flies (*Cantharis vittata*) collected as a substitute for Spanish flies (*Cantharis vesicatoria*), a blistering agent imported from Europe. Newspaper advertisements stated that gathering was best accomplished by "shaking the insects from the plants into hot water" and then drying them in the sun. Medical Purveyor James T. Johnson in Charlotte offered a "liberal price per pound," whereas Chisolm in Columbia promised two dollars per pound. Chemist Joseph LeConte, at the Columbia laboratory, reported using animal horns and bones to manufacture ammonia.[16]

Moore was dismayed by mistakes in a notice for indigenous plants issued by Medical Purveyor Richard Potts. "This publication with the many mistakes upon its face some of which are quite serious," he observed, "is evidently not at all creditable to a Med Officer. . . . You are instructed to be particular in seeing that the proper parts of Med Plants etc. are collected. In this connection it is stated for your information that the portion of the Podophyllum employed is the root and not the leaves or plant, which you advertise for, the latter being poisonous. You are directed for the future to be more particular in attending to such matters." Not only did this admonishment display the surgeon general's usual intolerance of sloppiness, but it also reflected detailed knowledge about the plants themselves.[17]

Moore was willing to try remedies not included in Porcher's book or in the 1863 *Standard Supply Table of the Indigenous Remedies*. When Medical Purveyor Chisolm forwarded to him a note from South Carolina physician J. A. Mayes suggesting that walnut-root bark could substitute for Spanish flies as a blistering agent, Moore ordered Surgeon James B. McCaw at Chimborazo Hospital to procure the bark and test its effectiveness.[18]

Underlying the use of indigenous plants was a friction between allopathic practitioners—the vast majority of Confederate surgeons—and various medical sects that objected to harsh methods and instead favored milder therapies often based on North American plants. Many allopaths considered sectarian practitioners to be quacks and were suspicious of their methods. Moore's intent was not to abandon allopathic therapy but to take advantage of remedies, derived from indigenous flora, that were unfamiliar to or previously underused by that practice. He nevertheless anticipated that his medical officers might misunderstand his motives. In the *Standard Supply Table of the Indigenous Remedies*, Moore wrote of the remedies: "It is hoped that Medical Officers will lay aside all prejudice which may exist in their minds against their use, and will give them a fair opportunity for the exhibition of those remedial virtues which they certainly possess."[19]

Knowing that most purveyors were not particularly knowledgeable about medicinal flora, the surgeon general hired W. T. Park, a sectarian physician of the "reform profession," to assist Prioleau in selecting and processing native plants. The medical purveyor was at first ignorant of how Moore intended for Park to assist, then became offended when they made decisions about which plants should receive priority in collecting. Disagreements between Prioleau and Park led to the latter leaving his position and accusing the former of poisoning the surgeon general's opinion against him. Writing of his duties assisting Prioleau, Park declared: "I admit I manifested a delight which might be construed by those of the opposite profession as an endeavor to promote the Reform Profession, when really my great aim and desire was for the relief of suffering humanity. Dr. Prioleau so construed it and reported me to the Surgeon General as endeavoring to promote the Reform Profession, and thereby arousing his antipathy to the Reform Profession and causing him to discontinue my agency."[20]

Moore's intense interest in indigenous flora extended to directing the movement of collected plant material between purveyors—a duty within the purview of Johns—providing new recipes for preparations, and researching the remedies' effectiveness. In December 1862 he instructed Prioleau: "You will forward to the Medical Director of the Department in which you are specimens of the various substances prepared for issue, requesting that they be submitted for trial to a few judicious and reliable medical officers in charge of hospitals who will be required to make to this office written reports as to their therapeutic value. Specimens will also be forwarded by you to this office through the purveyor in this city for the same purpose, all formulae used in the preparation of the indigenous extracts and tinctures being at the same time transmitted by mail."[21]

Moore said after the war that no indigenous remedies were found to be adequate substitutes for quinine, which was used primarily for malaria, or for opium, which was used primarily as an analgesic and antidiarrheal. One potential quinine substitute that particularly intrigued the surgeon general was Georgia bark (*Pinckneya pubens*). Moore was eager to learn of Prioleau's efforts, which turned out to be unsuccessful, to extract the plant's active ingredient. Probably the most common substitute for quinine was the compound tincture of indigenous barks, which was made by soaking the barks of dogwood, willow, and tulip poplar in whiskey. According to Moore, the unavailability of a good quinine substitute led to his instructing selected surgeons to test the subcutaneous injection of quinine, which required much smaller doses than those given orally, the standard route of administration.[22]

The surgeon general instructed his purveyors to publish notices urging ladies to grow opium poppies and collect the raw opium for delivery to them. C. B. Farmer of Walterboro, South Carolina, harvested opium "sufficient to supply his family and plantation negroes" for a year and promised to provide some of his excess harvest to Medical Purveyor Chisolm. Some growers in the South raised poppies for professional use by physicians or for profit, and it is possible that the Medical Department purchased opium from such ventures. Moore stated after the war that additional cultivation was attempted in

North Carolina—a possible reference to the efforts of Surgeon Aaron Snowden Piggot at Lincolnton—but yielded a small return, while two unsuccessful attempts were made "away down the Suwanee river" (which runs from southern Georgia into Florida). Shortly after the war, Northern physician and drug manufacturer Edward R. Squibb said: "I have heard that the culture of opium was attempted in Alabama and in Florida, in the neighborhood of Apalachicola, to a considerable extent. It was found to be deleterious to the field hands, and was abandoned on that account in some localities. That large quantities were produced, seems to be indisputable."[23]

The March 1862 pamphlet *General Directions for Collecting and Drying Medicinal Substances of the Vegetable Kingdom* recommended the collection of "inspissated juice of the garden lettuce" as a possible substitute for opium. The substance—known formally as lactucarium and informally as "lettuce opium"—was said in 1860 to be "highly esteemed by some, pronounced unreliable by others, and wholly neglected by the large majority of physicians." Some medical purveyors advertised for lettuce juice in 1862, but it did not appear in the *Standard Supply Table of the Indigenous Remedies* and seems not to have been collected or used to a large extent.[24]

Manufacturing Standard Medicines

The surgeon general had more than indigenous remedies in mind when he established the medical laboratories. In February 1865, Moore described the laboratories as not only preparing indigenous remedies, but having "been engaged more especially in the manufacture of [standard allopathic] medicines heretofore universally procured from abroad." Surviving records do not indicate the laboratories' relative production of standard versus indigenous medicines, but having the facilities devote attention to both may have reflected a realization that native remedies, by themselves, were not meeting the army's needs.[25]

Moore and his laboratory directors evidently concluded that some premade formulations that were not available on the market in adequate amounts, or that were exorbitantly priced, could be produced more economically in Confederate laboratories. Mercurial-pill mass, also called "blue mass," was a widely used preparation that always contained elemental mercury but could differ in its other components. Purveyor Chisolm, at his medical laboratory at Columbia, manufactured blue mass from imported mercury and other ingredients—powdered licorice root, powdered ginseng, honey, confection of roses, and rose petals—that were probably of domestic origin. He used newspapers to announce the need for rose petals, which were certainly intended for making blue mass. Mercury was just one example of an imported ingredient appearing in a medicine manufactured by a Confederate medical laboratory. Others included buchu (from southern Africa), colocynth (from Asia and Africa), and cubebs (from the East Indies), which were each made into extracts or fluid extracts.[26]

Moore realized that manufacturing standard medicines could require ingredients that were themselves difficult to procure. He approved the hiring of physician, chemist, and geologist Aaron Snowden Piggot and allowed him to establish a medical laboratory at a site of his choice—Piggot settled on Lincolnton, North Carolina—and to be free, to the extent possible, of the commercial aspects of being a medical purveyor. One of Piggot's major tasks was to use local mineral resources, such as iron pyrite and sulfur, in the manufacture of sulfuric acid, which itself was needed for the production of the anesthetics chloroform and ether. He also produced opiate preparations from poppies cultivated near his laboratory. Other medicinally useful plants cultivated at his direction included flax (for flaxseed and linseed oil), sorghum (for rum), and possibly black mustard.[27]

Black oxide of manganese, lime, Epsom salts, and alum were also mined, while potassium sulfate was salvaged from the Nitre and Mining Bureau as a byproduct of the manufacture of saltpeter, a constituent of gunpowder; all of these chemicals had medicinal use. Surgeon Chisolm needed silver to produce silver nitrate, so he published notices announcing his eagerness to pay for items containing the metal, including silver plate and silver spoons.[28]

Confederate medical laboratories represented an aggressive campaign to take advantage of the South's native flora as expedient substitutes for preferred conventional agents. Their production of conventional medicines indicated the surgeon general's preference to avoid the high prices of imported drugs and the fact that indigenous remedies were never meant to supplant their conventional counterparts.

With the exception of trading across enemy lines, which was not pursued aggressively enough to suit Surgeon General Moore, the means by which the Medical Department procured supplies were conducted with improvisation and vigor. Circumstances beyond the control of the department—an increasingly effective blockade, competition from other buyers, and the lack of a robust preexisting industrial base, for example—contributed to those methods being less than fully effective.

8. ✤ Care on and near the Battlefield

T he First Battle of Manassas, on July 21, 1861, was an early test of whether the Medical Department, still being organized at the time by Acting Surgeon General DeLeon, was up to the task of caring for large numbers of wounded soldiers. In their reports of the battle, Confederate commanders praised the performance of their medical officers, but the lack of an efficient system for the evacuation and treatment of the wounded was clear. Injured soldiers had to make their own way to aid stations, depend on their comrades to help take them there, or remain on the field and hope that someone would eventually retrieve them. The battle was also an indicator of what would be a chronic problem: a shortage of ambulance wagons. Deficiencies in battlefield care and evacuation were recognized widely enough that Richmond citizens, on the afternoon after the battle, agreed to dispatch a committee to Manassas to confer with the commanding generals about how to remove and transport the wounded.[1]

The army generally was unprepared for a large-scale war, while the Medical Department, in particular, had little direct control at first over how battlefield casualties were handled. Confederate army regulations on the topic were copied almost verbatim from the 1857 US Army regulations and did not change appreciably during the war except for reducing the number of ambulance and supply wagons allowed per unit. They assigned to the division quartermaster the responsibility for "all necessary arrangements for the transportation of the wounded," including placement of ambulance depots (temporary or movable hospitals) at convenient places behind the lines, where the wounded would be taken for treatment. "Active ambulances" would follow the troops to render immediate care to the wounded and remove them, by unspecified means, to the depots for further treatment. The division medical director, after consultation with the division quartermaster, would distribute his personnel as needed among the temporary hospitals and active ambulances and take his post at the principal depot. Establishment of hospitals "on the flanks or rear of the army" fell to the army's quartermaster general. These would receive patients, again by unspecified means, from the depots. Charles Smart, who served during the Civil War as a Union surgeon, criticized the 1857 regulations in comments that referred to the Union army but held equally well for its Confederate counterpart. The regulations, he said, reduced the status of the surgeon to "mere attendant on the wounded when permitted by the officers of another department [the quartermaster] to come into personal contact with them." Tying the medical director to the principal depot, said Smart, made that officer "a director only in name." Regulations thus made surgeons "responsible before public opinion for the care of the wounded, yet unable to accomplish anything without the consent and active cooperation of [Quartermaster Department] officers who were not held to this responsibility."[2]

The regulations described in vague terms the basic operation of the *ambulance volante* (flying ambulance) system of the French army, which originated during the Napoleonic Wars and is credited to French surgeons Dominique Jean Larrey and Pierre-François Percy. "As to the value and importance of such a system," wrote a contributor known only as "J.L.C." to a Southern newspaper in May 1861, "all army Surgeons and members of the professions are pretty well agreed, particularly in Europe, where they have been adopted, and carried out to an admirable degree of perfection." The French system would probably have been familiar to career American military physicians and to civilian practitioners as well: Larrey's memoirs were available in English translations, and his and Percy's innovations were described in British periodicals. In short, the system called for an ambulance corps that would establish aid stations, called ambulance depots, somewhat behind the battle line and send medical officers, assistants, and light wagons—the conglomeration constituting the flying ambulances—into the field with the troops. Personnel, equipped with stretchers, would immediately retrieve and treat the wounded as the men fell and use the light wagons to transport them to the depots, where they could receive further treatment and be removed to more permanent hospitals. Success of the system relied, in part, on having a highly organized corps of trained men and a sufficient number of ambulance wagons of appropriate design. Given the Confederacy's hurry to amass an army, the lack of military experience among most of its soldiers, and general shortcomings in equipping the troops, it is not surprising that an ineffective ambulance system would number among the "certain inevitable results of hasty and insufficient preparation and provisioning."[3]

Moore's Early Ideas on Medical Evacuation

Moore, on being appointed acting surgeon general, wasted little time in encouraging changes in the way the wounded were treated and removed from the battlefield. On August 19, 1861, he asked Secretary of War Walker to be notified of an impending action so that he could direct a reserve corps of operating surgeons, which did not exist at the time, to the battlefield. He also asked that various noncombatants accompanying regiments—including musicians, servants, and barbers—be organized into groups stationed with litters behind the line of battle. Those groups would quickly convey the wounded to ambulance wagons and awaiting surgeons; some of the individuals would carry emergency medical supplies and remain near the surgeons. Walker quickly approved the suggestions but said that "the chief difficulty . . . in reducing them to practice, would be found in the impossibility of giving the requisite notice of even the probable approach of a battle." Nevertheless, he told Moore that "some such arrangement . . . the details of which are left to your judgment, is recommended for your adoption, as far as may be practicable," especially for General Lee (commanding forces in Virginia) and Brigadier General Theophilus H. Holmes (commanding forces at Fredericksburg).[4]

Regulations and legislation at the time did not allow for a reserve corps of surgeons, but Moore had reason to hope that the situation would soon change. On the same day that he wrote to Walker (August 19), the Provisional Congress passed a bill to authorize the appointment of an additional assistant surgeon to each regiment in the army. Having two rather than one assistant surgeon per regiment might allow the formation of the reserve corps that Moore envisioned. President Davis had previously told William Porcher Miles, chairman of the Committee on Military Affairs, that the bill needed to be rephrased because it confused the regular with the provisional army and was unclear about whether the appointment of an additional assistant surgeon was mandatory rather than discretionary. Secretary Walker, who did not see the same problems, informed the president that congressional sentiment strongly favored the bill and recommended letting it pass unopposed. On August 22 Davis vetoed the bill on the grounds that previous legislation allowed the appointment of as many medical officers as necessary and that the mandatory addition of an assistant surgeon per regiment would be too costly. He added that complaints about medical care were more closely tied to surgeons' neglect or incompetence rather than inadequate numbers and that proper examination of surgeons would mitigate the problem. An attempt to override the veto failed.[5]

On December 14 Moore, evidently dissatisfied with these developments, sent Congressman Miles a letter (see Appendix C) explaining "a sketch of a Bill" that he hoped would enable his evacuation plan. The plan called for supernumerary medical officers and other personnel to staff highly portable temporary field hospitals, which he called "ambulances" in deference to the French, whose system he acknowledged emulating. After timely notification that a military engagement was imminent, brigades or divisions would establish field hospitals (ambulance depots) behind the lines. Regimental surgeons would not be detached from their units. Instead, supernumerary ambulance surgeons and soldier-nurses equipped with stretchers and medical supplies would follow troops into the field in wagons, tend to the wounded immediately, and send those needing further treatment to the nearest ambulance depot by stretcher or wagon. There the most experienced practitioners would handle the most complex cases; regimental surgeons would report to the depots, when able, to assist. Patients needing evacuation to fixed hospitals in the rear would be placed in spring wagons, accompanied by one or more ambulance surgeons, and taken to such facilities or to a railroad depot for transport to a general hospital elsewhere. The ambulance surgeons could, said Moore, assist on the battlefield before they were needed in the field hospitals and could even fill in at other times for regimental surgeons who were sick, injured, or otherwise unable to perform their duties. Congressional approval was needed, he told Miles, because current laws did not provide for medical officers other than regimental or hospital surgeons. Implementing the plan, said Moore, would require approval for a number of staff (as opposed to regimental or hospital) surgeons and assistant surgeons and a corps of military nurses.[6]

Moore's Modified Plan

The communication to Miles resulted in no immediate legislation, so Moore instituted various features of his plan anyway on May 7, 1862, through the issuance of a circular approved by the secretary of war, who by then was George W. Randolph. The circular accounted for personnel limits and the continuing shortage of ambulance and other wagons. Moore omitted the supernumerary surgeons he had previously described and called for "infirmary soldiers" to be detailed from the line by the commanding general. Regimental assistant surgeons, accompanied by infirmary soldiers, would follow their regiments into the field (not necessarily in wagons) and retrieve and tend to the wounded; patients requiring further treatment would be carried by stretcher (wagons were not mentioned as an option) to the nearest field infirmary (the term "ambulance depot" was dropped). Regimental surgeons would station themselves at the infirmaries, operate on or otherwise treat the wounded, and direct the removal of serious cases in wagons or carts (not necessarily accompanied by a surgeon) to fixed hospitals in the rear or to predetermined railroad depots or steamer landings for transportation to more remote general hospitals. The medical director would have overall charge of the infirmaries, operate on patients himself if necessary, and consult with other medical officers about the advisability of major surgery in specific cases. The instructions in Moore's circular resembled and were more thorough than those issued about a month earlier by Surgeon Edwin S. Gaillard, medical director of the Aquia District (part of the Department of Northern Virginia), and approved by the district commander, Major General Gustavus W. Smith. Whether Gaillard and Moore had previously discussed an ambulance system is unknown, but the former clearly believed that he could not wait for action from Congress or the surgeon general before taking organizational steps himself. Instructions similar to Gaillard's had also been issued, in March 1862, in the Army of the Mississippi, possibly at the suggestion of that army's medical director, Andrew Jackson Foard.[7]

Reports from the Seven Days' Battles (June 25–July 1, 1862) about Moore's new ambulance and infirmary system were largely positive, with commanders saying that wounded soldiers were "borne from the field as rapidly as they could be found" or "moved from the field, their wounds dressed and cared for, and all sent to the hospitals in the early morning." Major General A. P. Hill commended "the ambulance corps and drivers . . . for their active and untiring exertions in bringing off the wounded," while Brigadier General Joseph R. Anderson praised the infirmary-corps system as "wisely conceived" and "as far as my observation extended, faithfully executed by the several details."[8]

Compliments notwithstanding, the Medical Department's work on the battlefields was assisted by a civilian group called the Richmond Ambulance Committee (or Corps). The organization, which formed in response to "the government having made absolutely no provision for attention to the wounded or their removal to places of safety," sent volunteers, wagons, and food to find, assist, and remove the wounded, starting at the Battle of Williamsburg (May 5, 1862) and including "every important battlefield of the war which has been accessible to it." That the Confederate ambulance system still left much to be desired was confirmed by Lafayette Guild, medical director of the Army of Northern Virginia, after the Seven Days' Battles. "The present impromptu ambulance system of this army requires radical changes," he wrote to Surgeon General Moore, "and it is to be hoped that the efforts now being made to improve the efficiency of this important branch of our service may be successful." Nevertheless, said Guild, despite not having enough surgeons and ambulance wagons, "nearly all the necessary operations were performed in the field infirmaries and the wounded rapidly conveyed to the general hospitals." At the Battle of Fredericksburg in December 1862, he thought that the Ambulance Committee would be most useful transporting patients from the railroad depot to general hospitals. "On the battle field," he said, "they will be in the way, besides being unnecessarily exposed." Some small measure of assistance was provided when the AIGO declared in general orders on August 23, 1862, that ambulances and wagons used for regimental medical supplies were reserved for and under the control of the Medical Department, even though the vehicles and their teams and drivers would continue to appear on quartermasters' returns.[9]

Moore's vision for an efficient ambulance system depended on key medical officers being informed of an army's imminent movements and thus knowing where to place their resources to be most helpful. Guild described a major difficulty, at least as it existed in the Army of Northern Virginia:

> The movement of the army cannot be anticipated by me for the General Commanding [Robert E. Lee] never discloses any of his plans to those around him. The ch[ie]f officers of the different depts of his army are ordered to prepare to move just before the army takes up its line of march, and everything is done hurriedly and mysteriously. Were it in my power to keep you advised of all our movements I would most certainly do so; for it would add greatly to the efficiency of the corps.[10]

Legislative Failures

Guild's allusion after the Seven Days' Battles to efforts to improve the ambulance system may have been a reference to proposed legislation that would put into effect certain plans that Surgeon General Moore had suggested in his December 1861 letter to Congressman Miles. Secretary of War Randolph, who had approved Moore's circular of May 7, 1862, sent a proposed bill, probably in late August or early September, to Surgeon Gaillard for that officer's feedback. Gaillard had been severely wounded during the Battle of Seven Pines (May 31–June 1), had an arm amputated, and had been subsequently praised in the highest terms as having "few, if any, equals as an administrative and executive medical officer." The proposal sent to Gaillard contained two elements relevant to the ambulance system; his having already devised a similar system in the Aquia District may have made him especially qualified to provide critical remarks. First, the bill called for each infantry or cavalry regiment to be assigned one surgeon and two assistant surgeons instead of the current allotment of one of each. Second, it called for the formation of an infirmary corps of fifty able-bodied men from each brigade in the field. This corps would be organized into companies of fifty men and commanded by one first lieutenant, one second lieutenant, two sergeants, and two corporals.[11]

Gaillard wrote back to Randolph on September 3 in full support of adding an assistant surgeon per regiment and opined that doing so would make unnecessary Moore's concept of portable hospitals. A competent medical director, he noted, if given three medical officers per regiment, could form his own ambulance or hospital train and allow each brigade to act as a unit. Gaillard regarded the proposed infirmary corps as imperative but thought it should be formed of soldiers unfit for field duty. It should not be directed by the commissioned and noncommissioned officers mentioned in the bill, he thought, but should instead by directed by assistant surgeons.[12]

On September 4 Randolph sent Congressman Miles copies of Gaillard's remarks, Moore's previous (December 1861) letter to Miles, and the bill's draft and urged that the House Committee on Military Affairs consider the bill as being "of the utmost importance to the well being of the army." Miles introduced the measure (H.R. 29) on September 16, and the House and Senate passed it on October 3 after making a few small changes.[13]

President Davis agreed with the aims of the act but vetoed it on October 13. Referring to the sections pertinent to the ambulance system, he pointed out that current laws allowed for the *appointment* of only one surgeon and one assistant surgeon per regiment plus additional officers for hospitals (all in the PACS). The law's provisions were insufficient to allow the *assignment* of a large number of additional medical officers to regiments since medical officers could not be assigned unless they were first appointed. Although Davis described the bill's section on the infirmary corps as being "designed to effect a most humane and desirable object," he noted correctly that it did not allow for additional medical officers or for the corps to be under any control of medical officers; it did not even indicate any fixed duties of the corps. The president ended his veto message by encouraging Congress to develop additional legislation to attain the desired goals.[14]

Accordingly, two more attempts at Medical Department legislation, one from each chamber, arose during the spring of 1863. The Senate bill (S. 80) was introduced on March 12, 1863, passed by that chamber on April 11 with little ado, and sent to the House for concurrence. Among its provisions was the addition to the Medical Department of an infirmary corps consisting of as many assistant surgeons as deemed necessary by the president, up to one for each regiment in the field. The corps would take charge of the sick and wounded in camps and field hospitals under such legislation as prescribed by the president, who would also appoint its members.[15]

In the meantime, on April 10 the House passed a revised version of the bill (H.R. 29) vetoed by President Davis the previous October. Now known as H.R. 35, it was reworded to remove Davis's objections. Among its provisions was the establishment of an infirmary corps, consisting of up to one surgeon per brigade and one assistant surgeon per regiment, which would "not be attached to the organization of troops" but would instead serve in the field or in field hospitals under such regulations as the secretary of war might prescribe.[16]

For reasons that are unclear, the House postponed a decision on S. 80, and the Senate Committee on Military Affairs recommended that H.R. 35 ought not to pass. Thus, the congressional session ended on May 1, 1863, with neither bill being approved by both chambers.[17]

The Reserve Surgical Corps

Having seen Congress fail to enact legislation providing the supernumerary surgeons he thought necessary, Surgeon General Moore looked to a source that might be able to spare the needed medical officers: general hospitals. Thus, on March 15, 1864, he ordered hospital medical directors to designate one "skillful and efficient operative Surgeon" for every 500 beds under their jurisdiction. The selected men were to be available for temporary duty on or near battlefields in the Reserve Surgical Corps to help care for casualties; this would free regimental surgeons to accompany their units should they advance. Assignments would be made consequent to consultation between medical directors in the field and those with hospitals, with Reserve Surgical Corps members to be in readiness to proceed to any point after receiving telegraphic or other notice. Members would equip themselves with surgical instruments and dressings and coordinate with civilian ambulance and relief organizations to provide patients with a sufficient amount of cooked food. This action was evidently a response to a similar and successful action taken in the Army of Tennessee.[18]

To Moore's thinking, the Reserve Surgical Corps must have been a poor alternative to his original concept of dedicated ambulance surgeons who would travel with the army. Whereas his proposal would have provided valuable helping hands during battle and even in camp or on the march, the stated benefit of the Reserve Surgical Corps was simply to allow regimental surgeons to advance with their units instead of staying behind to care for their wounded. The failure of Congress to secure the appointment of additional medical officers for field service, either as supernumerary or regimental surgeons, forced Moore to take the needed doctors from hospitals, and the swiftness with which those men could arrive where needed could certainly not compare with having ambulance surgeons constantly on hand. His directive for Reserve Corps surgeons to work with civilian relief agencies such as the Richmond Ambulance Committee was an admission that the government could not be relied upon to adequately provide for its wounded soldiers.

To Medical Director of Hospitals William A. Carrington, Moore's directive did not adequately provide the reserve surgeons with medical supplies. He thus assigned a surgeon to act as medical purveyor for the Reserve Corps—composed of forty-two officers in April 1864—and asked Surgeon Johns, medical purveyor for Richmond, to furnish for that group supplies to be kept in Richmond and at a building in Gordonsville, Virginia. Carrington also asked him to "order or induce two of your most efficient packers or helpers" to accompany the supplies to Gordonsville when the corps was called out and to remain there as needed to assist the organization's medical purveyor. He feared the potentially large numbers of casualties from what would come to be called the Overland Campaign of Lieutenant General Ulysses S. Grant. Thus, on May 24, 1864, Carrington urged Moore to temporarily detach one medical officer from each regiment to be assigned to the Reserve Corps or to accompany wounded soldiers to the rear. This suggestion must have struck the surgeon general as ironic in light of his past efforts to enlarge the regimental allotment of medical officers from two to three. Carrington explained that "the ravages of battle have thinned out the regiments so that one med. officer can easily perform all the duties required, especially when regiments are brigaded and arrangements made by the Reserve Corps and Ambulance Committee to care for the wounded." Carrington provided the example of a regiment with three medical officers, one of whom "had been brigade surgeon . . . and is I understand generally detached from regimental duty though contrary to all orders on the subject." Because a senior surgeon of brigade, as Carrington noted, was supposed to retain his regimental duties, his regiment would not be entitled to another (third) medical officer.[19]

Ongoing Problems

In addition to lacking the necessary human resources—regimental or supernumerary surgeons—to help staff the ambulance system he envisioned, Surgeon General Moore was also much hampered by the aforementioned ambulance shortage. Medical Department regulations in 1861 called for a regiment to have two four-wheeled ambulances, ten two-wheeled ambulances, and four two-wheeled transport carts for supplies. Starting in 1862, revised regulations set the regimental allowance at two four-wheeled and two two-wheeled ambulances and one wagon for supplies. Surgeon J. J. Chisolm reported that four-wheeled ambulances (spring wagons) were generally used by Confederate forces, although two-wheeled vehicles were also to be seen. The original 1861 allowance, he observed, was never actually delivered, and a regiment typically had just one supply wagon and one (rarely two) four-wheeled ambulance. Chisolm seemed to put the blame on the Quartermaster Department for not supplying an adequate number of suitable vehicles. "Could those in the quartermaster's department," he said, "undergo the same treatment which falls to the lot of the sick and wounded during transportation, there would be a few more comforts extended to those who are periling their lives for their country's safety."[20]

The Quartermaster Department operated a shop in Richmond—located on the south dock, across from Libby Prison—that manufactured 264 ambulance wagons in 1864, but the total extent to which the Confederate government produced such vehicles is unclear. Purchases and captures also contributed to the supply of ambulances.[21]

Moore's vision of an ambulance and evacuation system—first expressed in rudimentary form in August 1861 and then more fully in December—resembled the one implemented by Surgeon Jonathan Letterman as medical director of the Union's Army of the Potomac in 1862 and later adopted by all Federal armies. The basic concepts behind each system were developed by the French decades earlier, and the success of his concept as adopted by the Union armies helped earn Letterman the sobriquet of "the father of battlefield medicine." Moore's hopes, on the other hand, were continually stymied by an insufficiency of surgeons and of ambulance wagons and by the failure of the Confederate Congress and President Davis to agree on legislation that would help bring the surgeon general's concepts to fruition. Energetic medical officers used available resources to improve medical evacuation markedly after the chaos of the First Battle of Manassas. They could not function at the same level as their better-supplied and supported Union counterparts, but this deficiency could not be attributed to a lack of energy or original thought on the part of Surgeon General Moore.[22]

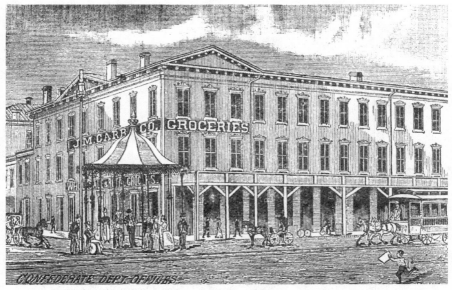

An 1885 view of the building at Commerce and Bibb Streets, Montgomery, Alabama, that housed the Confederate War Department and other government offices until June 1861. *H. G. McCall,* A Sketch, Historical and Statistical, of the City of Montgomery *(Montgomery, AL: W. D. Brown, 1885).*

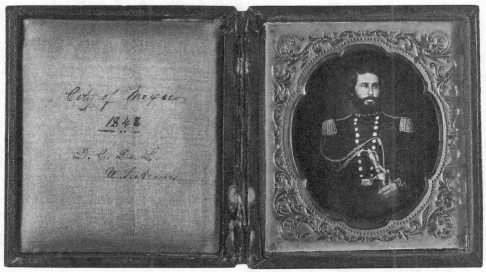

David Camden DeLeon as a US medical officer during the Mexican War, 1848. De-Leon was the first acting surgeon general of the Confederate army. The inscription is not in DeLeon's handwriting. © *Stanley B. Burns, MD, and The Burns Archive.*

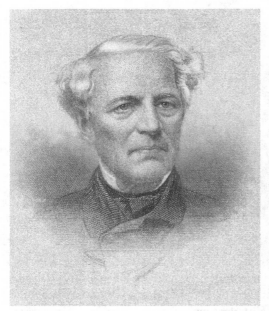

Samuel Cooper, adjutant and inspector general of the Confederate army. Cooper was the highest-ranking officer in the army and a confidant of President Jefferson Davis. *Engraving by John A. O'Neill (New York: C. B. Richardson, 1865[?]). Author's collection.*

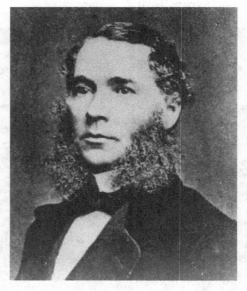

Samuel Preston Moore, surgeon general of the Confederate army through most of the Civil War. Moore's disciplined management style contributed to the efficiency of the Medical Department. *Courtesy of the Waring Historical Library, Medical University of South Carolina, Charleston.*

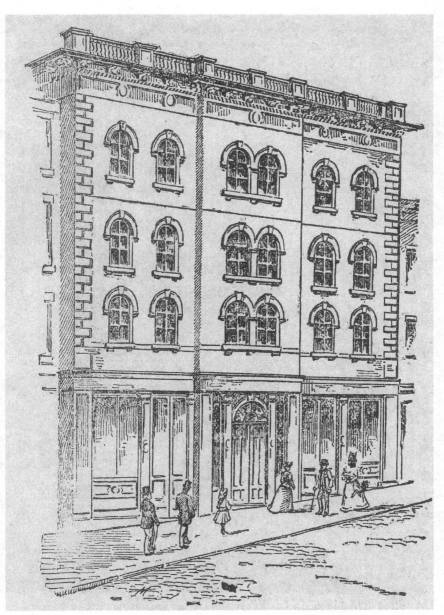

The Virginia Mechanics Institute building on Ninth Street, opposite Bank Street, in Richmond. The structure housed the Confederate Surgeon General's Office (SGO) and other War Department and government offices from July 1861 through the end of the war. It was destroyed in the fire of April 1865. Richmond Dispatch, *June 30, 1896*.

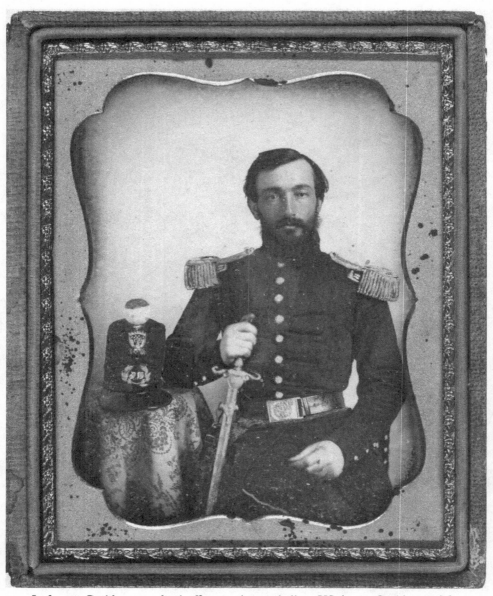

Lafayette Guild as a medical officer in the antebellum US Army. Guild served for most of the Civil War as medical director of the Confederate Army of Northern Virginia. *American Civil War Museum, under the management of the Virginia Museum of History and Culture, Richmond (FIC2009.0151).*

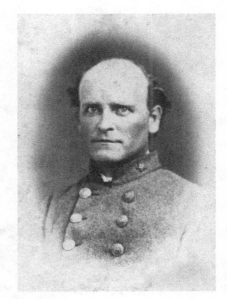

Surgeon Samuel H. Stout, superintendent of hospitals and later medical director
of hospitals for the Confederate Army of
Tennessee. *Virginia Museum of History and
Culture, Richmond (1990.100.466).*

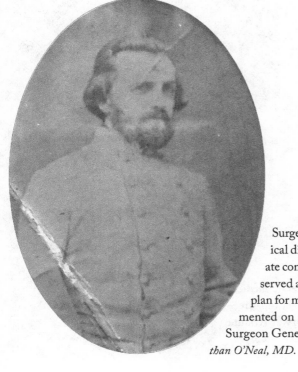

Surgeon Edwin S. Gaillard, medical director of various Confederate commands. Gaillard, who also
served as an inspector, developed a
plan for medical evacuation and commented on a similar plan proposed by
Surgeon General Moore. *Courtesy of Jonathan O'Neal, MD.*

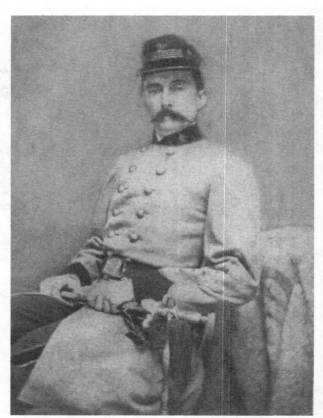

Surgeon Thomas H. Williams, an early medical director of the Army of Northern Virginia. In the latter half of the war, Williams served in the SGO, in charge of medical purveying. *Roberts, "Confederate Medical Service."*

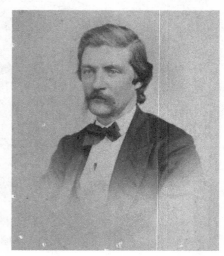

George S. Blackie, Confederate medical purveyor for northern Georgia and director of the medical laboratory at Atlanta (later moved to Augusta). *Courtesy of Jonathan O'Neal, MD.*

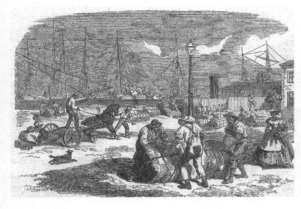

Workers at Nassau, the Bahamas, unloading cotton from blockade-runners newly arrived from Southern ports. The vessels would return to the South with European goods, while the cotton would be sent to Europe on larger vessels. Illustrated London News, *April 30, 1864.*

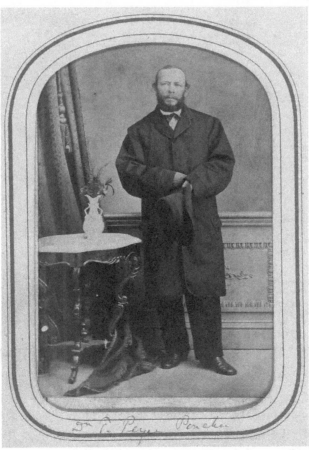

Physician and botanist Francis Peyre Porcher, who served as a Confederate surgeon and wrote *Resources of the Southern Fields and Forests. Courtesy of the South Caroliniana Library, University of South Carolina, Columbia.*

Confederate States of America.

MEDICAL PURVEYOR'S OFFICE,

Savannah, September 8th. 1862.

The following named Indigenous Remedies are wanted by the Medical Department, for which the annexed prices will be paid. To be delivered at either of my Offices in Savannah or Macon, properly dried and in good order, labeled, and each, when practicable, containing a dried specimen of the whole plant.

	Per Pound.		Per Pound.
Arum Triphyllum, Root, (Indian Turnip, or Wake Robin)	$ 30	Iris Versicolor, root, (Blue Flag,)	30
Asclepias Tuberosa, Root, (Pleurisy or Butterfly Weed Root)	25	Juglans Cinerea, leaves and inner bark of root, (Butternut,)	50
Aristolochia Serpentaria, Root, (Virginia Snake Root)	1 00	Lobelia Inflata, seeds, (Lobelia)	1 50
Arctostaphylos Uva Ursi, Leaves, (Uva Ursi)	30	" " herb, "	50
Arctium Lappa, Root, (Burdock)	20	Leptandra Virginica, root, (Black Root, Culver's Physic)	50
" " Seeds, "	20	Laurus Sassafras, red, bark of root, (Sassafras)	30
Asarum Canadense, Root, (Wild Ginger or Colts Foot, &c.)	50	Liquidambar Styraciflua, inner bark, (Sweet Gum Tree)	10
Apocynum Androsemifolium, Root, (Bitter Root)	40	" " resin, " "	1 00
" Cannabinum, Root, (Indian Hemp)	50	Myrica Cerifera, bark of root, (Low Bush Myrtle)	35
Acorus Calamus, root, (Calamus)	25	Mentha Piperita, herb, (Peppermint)	30
Cimicifuga Racemosa, root, (Black Cohosh)	50	" Viridis, " (Spearmint)	25
Corallorhiza Odontorhiza, root, (Crawley)	2 00	Nymphea Odorata, root, (White Pond Lilly)	10
Cypripedium Pubescens, root, (Lady's Slipper)	1 00	Polygala Senega, root, (Seneca Snake Root)	1 00
Convallaria Multiflora, root, (Solomon's Seal)	30	Prunus Virginiana, bark, (Wild Cherry Tree)	30
Corydalis Formosa, root, (Turkey Corn, Wild Turkey Pea)	50	Podophyllum Peltatum, root, (Mandrake)	30
Chionanthus Virginica, bark of root, (Fringe Tree)	30	Panax Quinquefolium, root, (Ginseng)	50
Chimaphila Umbellata, whole plant, (Pipssewa)	30	Pinckneya Pubens, inner bark,	30
Chelone Glabra, leaves and small twigs, (Balmony)	50	Phytolacca Decandra, berries, (Poke)	30
Conium Maculatum, leaves and seeds, (Poison Hemlock)	25	Rhus Glabra, berries, (Sumach Berries)	15
Chenopodium Anthelminticum, seeds, (Jerusalem Oak)	25	Ricinus Communis, seeds, (Palma Christi) per bushel	7 00
Capsicum of all kinds, (Red Pepper)	1 00	Sanguinaria Canadensis, root, (Blood Root) per pound	50
Euphorbia Ipecacuanha, bark of root, (Wild Ipecac)	50	Symphytum Officinale, root, (Comfrey)	25
Eupatorium Perfoliatum, small twigs, leaves and flowers.		Sinapis Alba, seeds, (White Mustard)	75
(Boneset)	30	" Nigra, " (Black Mustard)	75
Eupatorium Purpurium, root, (Queen of the Meadow,)	50	Stillingia Sylvatica, root, (Queens Delight)	20
Geranium Maculatum, root, (Cranesbill or Crowfoot)	1 00	Salix, inner bark, (Willow)	30
Gelseminum Sempervirens, root, (Yellow Jessamine)	25	Spigelia Marilandica, root, (Pink Root)	30
Hyoscyamus Nigra, leaves and seeds, (Henbane)	50	Ulmus Fulva, inner bark (Slippery Elm)	30
Hydrastis Canadensis, root, (Golden Seal,)	1 00	Veratrum Viride, root, (American Hellebore)	25
Hamamelis Virginica, leaves, (Witch Hazel)	30	Xanthoxylum Fraxineum, bark, (Prickly Ash)	30
" " bark of shrub, "	30	" " berries, "	50

W. H. PRIOLEAU,

Ass't Surg. P. A. C. S., and Medical Purveyor 4th Depot.

Handbill calling on Southern citizens to gather medicinal plants for sale to the Medical Department. *Entry 30, RG 109, National Archives and Records Administration, Washington, DC.*

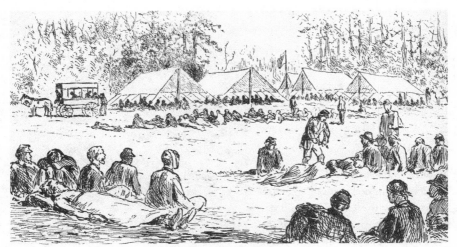

Illustration of a Confederate field hospital, by Edwin Forbes. A four-wheeled ambulance is next to the tents. *George F. Williams,* Bullet and Shell: War as the Soldier Saw It *(New York: Fords, Howard, and Hulbert, 1882).*

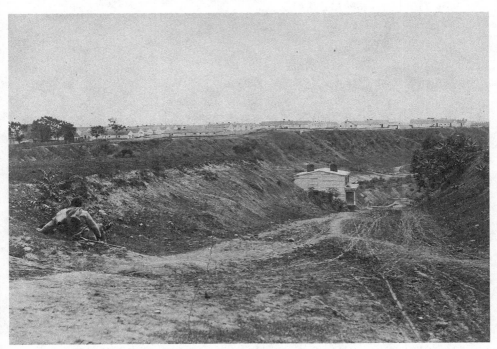

The pavilion-style Chimborazo Hospital, built on a plateau just east of the Richmond city limits. The facility eventually consisted of about 150 buildings supplemented by tents. *Library of Congress (reprod. no. LC–DIG–ppmsca–33629).*

Confederate surgeon Joseph Jones, who was assigned to investigate disease during the Civil War and described the horrid conditions at the Andersonville prison camp. *Joseph Jones Papers, Louisiana Research Collection, Tulane University Special Collections, Howard-Tilton Memorial Library, Tulane University, New Orleans.*

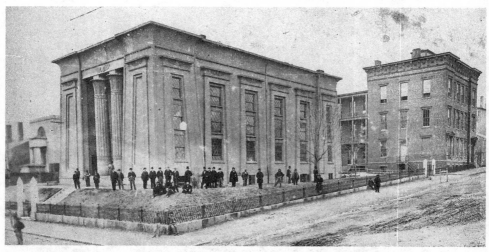

The Medical College of Virginia (MCV), one of the few Southern medical schools that remained open throughout the Civil War. Among its students were Confederate hospital stewards training to become medical officers. MCV also hosted wartime meetings of the Association of Army and Navy Surgeons. At the right is the MCV Hospital, which treated Confederate soldiers. *Special Collections and Archives, Tompkins-McCaw Library, Virginia Commonwealth University, Richmond.*

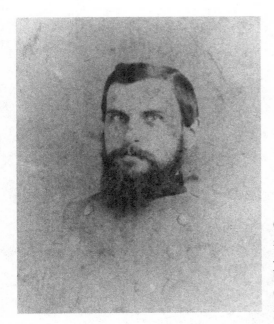

Confederate surgeon J. J. Chisolm, medical purveyor and author of *A Manual of Military Surgery*. His book went through three editions during the Civil War. *Courtesy of the J. J. Chisolm family.*

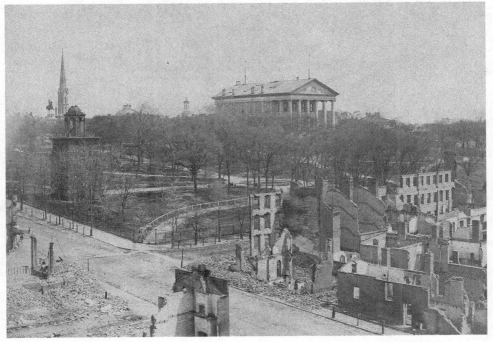

Richmond's Capitol Square shortly after the fire of April 1865. The ruins of the Virginia Mechanics Institute building, which housed the Medical Department, are just above the lower left corner of this cropped image. *Photograph by Hathaway. The Valentine, Richmond.*

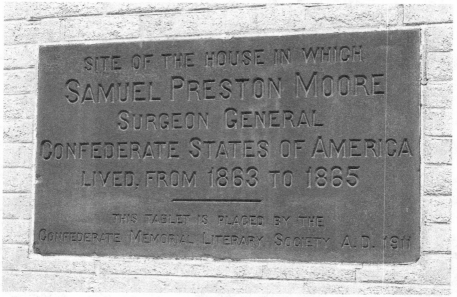

Tablet originally placed in 1911 to identify a wartime residence of Surgeon General Moore in Richmond. It is now on an exterior wall of the Richmond Police Headquarters building at the northwest corner of West Grace and North Jefferson Streets. *Photograph by the author.*

9. ❄ General Hospitals

After sick and wounded soldiers received treatment on the battlefield or in regimental or field hospitals, those requiring additional care were moved to larger permanent or semipermanent facilities at some distance from the front lines, there to convalesce or to receive more definitive treatment. The term "general hospitals" was commonly used at the time to describe such facilities and was derived, according to historian H. H. Cunningham, from their practice of not restricting admission to soldiers of particular units. Derivation notwithstanding, it is useful to apply a distinction used by Medical Director of Hospitals William A. Carrington. He understood "that a regimental or field hospital is a temporary organization either in tents or buildings previously existing, that are immediately attached to the troops in the field, and that only the cases that require separation from other troops for a few days should be admitted into them, and the medical officers and attendants are temporarily detailed from the Regts." On the other hand, Carrington saw general hospitals as "intended for more permanent occupation—near or far from the army in proportion to the facility of transportation" and "more complex in organization." These were larger operations than regimental hospitals, had their own dedicated staff, and received patients from more than one regiment, although many were designated for soldiers of particular states. How general hospitals were to be organized and who was to operate them vexed the Medical Department from the start, when officials had no way to predict the length and severity of the war. Consequently, early government preparations were inadequate for the large numbers of soldiers becoming ill in camp or who would be wounded in upcoming battles.[1]

Initial Preparations

In the mid-nineteenth century, patients who required medical care and had adequate financial means were usually seen in their home by a physician and nursed by family members. Hospitals, established by county or municipal organizations or by private groups, cared for the indigent and for patients with mental illness. When the Civil War broke out, Richmond, which would become the South's major hospital center, had five relatively small hospitals, none of which were then operated by the Confederate government or intended for soldiers. There was no expectation—at least at the time—that the Confederate government would take sole responsibility for the care of sick or wounded soldiers.[2]

Thus, existing hospitals began preparing for military patients, and citizens and civic groups started making arrangements for additional facilities even before the first major combat of the war at Manassas, Virginia. In Richmond, for example, the Infirmary of St. Francis de Sales, operated by the Sisters of Charity, was declared ready to receive military patients on May 3, 1861. During the same month, Alabamian Juliet Opie Hopkins took steps to establish a hospital in Richmond for Alabama soldiers. Also in June, Letitia Tyler Semple, a daughter of former president John Tyler, used her father's influence to obtain permission from the secretary of war to establish a hospital in Williamsburg, Virginia. There was a need for soldiers' hospitals even in the absence of combat since troops became ill in camp, where crowding contributed to disease. Particularly vulnerable were troops from rural areas, who contracted illnesses, such as measles and mumps, that their city-raised comrades had experienced as children but could have more serious consequences in adults. Lax sanitary practices and poorly prepared food contributed to the frequent occurrence of diarrhea and dysentery. Richmond's Company G Hospital, established by neighborhood citizens, was reported on June 1 to be caring for fifty or sixty ill soldiers, mostly from a Tennessee regiment. On about that date in the same part of town, the Masons' Hall Hospital received thirty-six sick soldiers from an Arkansas regiment. Although patients in those facilities would presumably be seen by a physician from time to time, their recovery, in the minds of the citizenry, would depend largely on attentive nursing care provided by women.[3]

Disease was also taking its toll elsewhere in the Confederacy. When Surgeon Samuel H. Stout arrived to take command of Nashville's Gordon Hospital in October, for example, he found some 650 patients lying in bunks or on the floor of the former warehouse. Most were suffering from measles or its complications. The hospital, then in charge of the Nashville Hospital Association, seemed disorganized, had no record books, and was attended by civilian physicians hired by the association.[4]

The individual states, or organizations supported by their governments, were eager to help care for their own soldiers. Rev. Robert W. Barnwell Jr., representing the South Carolina Hospital Aid Association, proposed to President Davis and Acting Surgeon General DeLeon on July 4—more than two weeks before the First Battle of Manassas—that citizens of South Carolina establish hospitals along the line of Confederate defenses. The facilities were envisioned as temporary and not "embarrassed by the technicalities incident to Governmental operations." Davis and DeLeon, according to Barnwell and his associates, deemed the plan "impracticable and promotive only of confusion and evil," incapable of promising "permanent relief," and "calculated to impede, rather than promote, the operations of the Medical Department of the Army." Although their concerns were not described more specifically, they likely centered on exactly the casual nature of operations that the South Carolinians anticipated: The hospitals would probably lack the government control, discipline, and strict recordkeeping of true military facilities. Such a state of affairs would probably have been antithetical to how the president and acting surgeon general—both well versed in military ways—imagined that such hospitals should function. For the time being, the South Carolina organization would have to be content with amassing supplies for distribution to hospitals treating the state's sick and wounded. But the Confederate government, which wanted to be, in the words of historian Frank E. Vandiver, a "model of decentralization and a bulwark of state sovereignty," could not forever dismiss the fact that "states wanted to care for their own men and no others."[5]

It is difficult to discern DeLeon's plans and actions for general hospitals, but First Manassas demonstrated an obvious unpreparedness for large numbers of casualties. The Richmond Alms House had been leased to Confederate authorities by the Richmond City Council, and the structure was established as a Confederate hospital on June 30, about two weeks before DeLeon was relieved as acting surgeon general. That facility took in Union soldiers wounded in the battle and was later converted to a general hospital for Confederate troops. In addition to the Infirmary of St. Francis de Sales, at least three of Richmond's other four prewar hospitals—the Main Street Hospital (previously used for slaves), Bellevue Hospital, and the MCV Hospital—admitted Confederate casualties from Manassas. It is unclear whether Richmond's fifth prewar hospital, City Hospital, treated soldiers wounded at Manassas, although it did admit soldiers later in the war. The Confederate wounded, once they filled the small number of preexisting hospital beds, were treated in private homes and other buildings, such as unoccupied wooden structures and tobacco factories.[6]

The procurement of the Richmond Alms House was not the only sign that Confederate officials were aware before First Manassas of shortcomings in their fledgling hospital system. Early on, attendant duties in general hospitals were typically performed by convalescing patients, who often lacked the requisite skills and temperament. Commanders were quick to suggest a remedy. Brigadier General John B. Magruder, commanding at Williamsburg and Yorktown, Virginia, noted on July 18 that "the troops here being Volunteers, and unused to such duties as are required from Hospital Attendants and nurses, cooks &c, the sick in the Hospitals suffer greatly, if left to their care." Black women, said Magruder, were entirely suitable for these tasks and could be hired for six dollars per month, half the pay of a soldier, and would free attendant troops for other duty. His letter made its way to the SGO, and Charles H. Smith, now temporarily in charge of the office, asked Secretary of War Walker on July 24 to suggest that the Provisional Congress introduce legislation authorizing appropriations to pay civilian cooks and nurses for hospitals. The SGO, said Smith, had received frequent communications suggesting such action. On August 7 Walker forwarded Smith's and Magruder's letters to William Porcher Miles, chairman of the Committee on Military Affairs, for that group's consideration. Miles, fellow South Carolinian Samuel Preston Moore—who had recently become acting surgeon general—and Secretary Walker quickly collaborated to draft a bill calling for an appropriation of $130,000 for such cooks and nurses. On August 15 President Davis asked congressmen to support the bill, which was passed on August 20 and signed by Davis on the twenty-first.[7]

Two other bills aimed at improving care in general hospitals were approved on August 21. One, which Secretary Walker urged the president to support, called for an appropriation for the hiring of civilian physicians (contract surgeons) to assist army surgeons. Again, Congressman Miles was supportive, and the bill, which appropriated $50,000, was passed by the Provisional Congress on August 20 and approved by President Davis that following day. Also on August 21, Davis approved a bill appropriating the curiously small sum of $50,000 for the establishment and support of military hospitals. Both appropriations were for the remainder of the fiscal year, which ended in February 1862.[8]

Additional discussion of the need for nurses occurred in the aftermath of First Manassas. On August 8 Acting Surgeon General Moore informed Secretary Walker that $22,000 would pay for nurses at the Confederacy's "large hospitals where the sick are congregated in large numbers." Those facilities were at Culpeper Court House, Manassas, Winchester, Staunton, Gordonsville, and Orange Court House, Virginia; within the commands of Brigadier General Magruder (District of Yorktown, Department of the Peninsula) and Brigadier General Benjamin Huger (Department of Norfolk); and at Pensacola, Florida.

In October 1861 Judah Benjamin, who had succeeded Walker as secretary of war, and President Davis ruled that hospital matrons—white women whose duties could range from administering medicines and dressing wounds to supervising hospitals' domestic operations—could be paid from the $50,000 appropriation for hospitals approved in August.[9]

Congressman William H. Macfarland, reporting on August 31 for a special committee appointed to examine the condition of hospitals, stated that those in Richmond were, by then, skillfully directed, generally in good condition, and adequately supplied and staffed. "It does not seem to the committee," he concluded," that any special legislation is now necessary."[10]

Allowing State Involvement

Despite Macfarland's rosy assessment, the inadequacy of existing hospitals evidently convinced Acting Surgeon General Moore and the War Department that it was no longer prudent to discourage state involvement in establishing general hospitals. Not only would state-sponsored hospitals provide more beds, but contributions to them by the states also would save money for the Confederate government, and soldiers would be comforted by being surrounded by caregivers and other patients from their own state. The Georgia Relief and Hospital Association was particularly effusive in December 1861 about the cooperation it was receiving from the SGO:

> The acting Surgeon general, Dr. S. P. Moore, has shown great discrim-
> ination and good judgment in recognizing, and giving encouragement
> to the establishment of State Hospitals in Virginia. . . . Thoroughly
> intelligent in all that relates to his important branch of the service, he
> has earnestly labored to secure a reliable and efficient organization.
> Any proposition, however unusual, which promised to improve the
> condition of the army was sure to meet his cordial co-operation. The
> offer of individual States and of State organizations to establish Hos-
> pitals in Virginia, though without precedent, was wisely and liberally
> encouraged.[11]

According to the association, the general understanding between individual states and the Confederate government acknowledged that state hospitals were established by and received considerable support from the states. The facilities, however, were to be operated as government hospitals under military authority, and their surgeons, preferably from the sponsoring state, were to be commissioned officers in the army. The Confederate government often hired contract surgeons to help staff the state hospitals and provided the facilities with rations; credit for rations not used would accumulate in a hospital fund that could be used to purchase special food items or other goods. The Georgia association established four hospitals in Richmond, the first opening on September 5, 1861, and the last on May 7, 1862.[12]

Among the state hospitals within or close to Richmond were one for Louisiana, which opened on September 4, 1861, and four for Alabama, the first of which opened on August 1, 1861. Most or all of the Alabama hospitals were organized by the aforementioned Juliet Opie Hopkins. The previously rebuffed South Carolina Hospital Aid Association, with the assistance of the Confederate surgeon in charge of hospitals in Charlottesville, Virginia, established a state hospital in that town and agreed with Acting Surgeon General Moore to organize additional facilities with terms similar to those given the Georgia Relief and Hospital Association. Moore apparently expressed "doubts of the advisability of a South Carolina hospital in Richmond," so in October 1861 that state's organization opened a hospital in the town of Manchester, just across the James River from the capital. The group opened additional Virginia hospitals in Warren Springs (November 1861), Charlottesville (December 1861), and Petersburg (April 1862). In November 1861 the South Carolina association also proposed to Surgeon Thomas H. Williams, medical director of the Confederate Army of the Potomac, the establishment of a hospital at Salem, Virginia. Williams replied that if the facility could not accommodate at least a hundred patients, it "would be of little benefit to the service" and "the project had better be abandoned," which it was.[13]

North Carolinians were quick to establish army hospitals in their own state for troops gathering there to organize and train. They also opened two state establishments in Petersburg, Virginia, in October 1861 and early 1862. A general hospital in Richmond and eventually designated for North Carolina soldiers was formed relatively late, in May or June 1862. Although it is commonly thought to have been established through efforts of the North Carolina Medical Department, period accounts suggest a more reactive role by the state. Otis F. Manson, a Virginia native who had lived in North Carolina since 1841, was serving as a medical officer in the Confederate army as early as April 1862. On June 1 he was appointed surgeon and assigned to a factory-turned-hospital at Twenty-Sixth and Main Streets in Richmond, which quickly became known as Moore Hospital (later General Hospital No. 24). "As I was the only Surgeon hailing from N.C. in charge of a hospital here [in Richmond]," said Manson in 1863, "it became filled with N.C. sick & wounded from its opening." Later in 1862 it was officially set apart for North Carolina troops. Edward Warren, surgeon general of North Carolina, reported in November 1864 that General Hospital No. 24 had "been regarded by the State as under her particular protection," having been paying rent for the property for more than a year and furnishing important supplies. The facility would later be a topic of contention between Surgeon General Moore and North Carolina officials.[14]

On January 29, 1862, a special committee of the Provisional Congress praised the "admirable manner" in which state-established hospitals were conducted, encouraged the Confederate government to emulate their level of care, and expressed gratitude for citizens' contribution to the well-being of patients. Nevertheless, the Medical Department's original apprehensions about nongovernment hospitals persisted. In September 1861, for example, a Richmond newspaper cited "serious questions whether it would not be better to suspend the private hospitals and to terminate the practice of taking sick soldiers into private houses, by an enlargement of the government hospitals, and a considerable increase of the medical staff on duty in Richmond." Indeed, a viewpoint shared by Moore and other senior medical officers was expressed by the newspaper when it observed that hospitals needed "a central organization competent to direct and control the whole matter without supplementary aids or unpleasant interferences with its authority.[15]

Pavilion Hospitals

Encouraging, or at least tolerating, state involvement after First Manassas was an expedient on Moore's part, but he recognized that the current state of Richmond hospitals was far from satisfactory. The structures—factories, warehouses, public buildings, and the like—being used to house sick and wounded soldiers presented numerous problems, "the principal being the liability of spreading contagious diseases among the inhabitants of the city; the aggregation of so many patients in the necessarily large wards of the factories, thereby contaminating the buildings, rendering them unfit for occupancy;

and the impossibility of supplying by these means the further demands of the service." Indeed, well-informed physicians believed that contagious diseases were spread through the atmosphere and that the gaseous emanations of the lungs and skin of sick (and even healthy) people, if not diluted sufficiently and continuously with fresh air, were unhealthful. Thus, it was vital for hospitals to avoid overcrowding, to maintain cleanliness, and to provide adequate ventilation. These principles were well known in the mid-nineteenth century, incorporated into the construction of new hospitals, and encouraged by nursing advocate and social reformer Florence Nightingale. Moore's concern about the future unavailability of contaminated buildings reflected the belief that such spaces should be emptied of patients and undergo the time-consuming process of vigorous cleaning, fumigation, and airing out.[16]

Moore consequently enlisted the help of physician James B. McCaw, a faculty member at MCV. Together, they determined that a plateau called Chimborazo Hill, just east of the Richmond city limits and designated as a site for winter quarters, would suit admirably for the construction of a pavilion-style hospital. That design, meant to incorporate the recommendations of Nightingale and others, consisted of numerous elongated, quickly built one-story wards, each of which had ample windows and other features to ensure adequate ventilation. The walls consisted of undressed vertical pine boards nailed onto wooden framing, with strips covering the gaps between boards. Rough planks constituted the floors, and the roofs were shingled. The compound, called Chimborazo Hospital, opened in October 1861 under the command of Surgeon McCaw. It would eventually have about 150 buildings, each with a capacity of forty to sixty patients; the structures were supplemented by tents. The complex was divided into five divisions (sometimes themselves called hospitals), each administered by a separate surgeon. That Moore and McCaw preferred the pavilion design is hardly surprising, given its familiarity to hospital experts and Nightingale's advocacy. In fact, the US Sanitary Commission recommended in July 1861 that Union military hospitals be built on the same plan, and Surgeon Charles S. Tripler, medical director of the Union Army of the Potomac, argued in September 1861 for the design in terms that Moore would probably endorse completely: "In my opinion, frame huts . . . are much better adapted to hospital purposes that large buildings of masonry, such as hotels, colleges, and the like. They admit of more perfect ventilation, can be kept in better police, are more convenient for the sick and wounded and their attendants, admit of a ready distribution of patients into proper classes, and are cheaper."[17]

Surgeon Francis Sorrel, who joined Moore's staff in August 1861, asserted that other Richmond pavilion hospitals, such as Winder, Howard's Grove, and Jackson, were organized under his own "personal care and supervision." The size and complexity of Chimborazo and Winder Hospitals resulted in their being designated military posts, with the commander of the Department of Henrico assigning them commandants and guards. Sorrel was dispatched in March 1862 to the headquarters of General Albert Sidney Johnston, commander of the Army of the Mississippi, "to organize hospitals in the rear of his army, extending to and including nearby towns and cities southward to the Gulf." Among his actions were instructing Surgeon Samuel H. Stout, then in Decatur, Alabama, to improve the "filthy" hospitals in Chattanooga, which had just been put in Stout's charge, and to send patients to better facilities established by Sorrel in Atlanta. He then returned to Richmond and was "put in charge of all the general hospitals east of the Mississippi."[18]

The construction of wood-framed pavilion hospitals of large capacity would allow many temporary hospitals to be closed, with only those in large factory buildings being kept if needed. It also made it easy and relatively inexpensive to abandon individual wards if necessary—because of contamination, for example. Yet "building and furnishing hospitals," said Moore after the war, "had to depend entirely upon the quartermaster and commissary departments, hence much delay was experienced in obtaining proper hospital accommodations, and in such cases blame was attached to the medical bureau which it never deserved." His assessment was not mere after-the-fact rationalizing. In April 1862 Moore explained that crowding in Richmond hospitals must exist "until the buildings being fitted are completed." In January 1864 he appealed to Lieutenant General Leonidas Polk, commanding the Department of Alabama, Mississippi, and East Louisiana—and apparently to other commanders—for assistance in appointing special quartermaster and commissary officers to assist in the organization and supply of hospitals. Moore's previous communications to the quartermaster general and commissary general on the topic, he informed Polk, had arrived at "no conclusion."[19]

It is unclear whether Moore had an ideal ward design in mind for pavilion hospitals, and, if so, whether he prescribed it in writing or through Surgeon Sorrel. The wards at Chimborazo were described as having four rows of bunks rather than the usually recommended two, but that configuration may have resulted from the hospital's use of barracks that were already in place and originally intended for winter quarters. Surgeon Stout, who was assigned responsibility for general hospitals in the Army of Tennessee, believed that wards wide enough to accommodate more than two rows of bunks could not provide adequate ventilation for patients in the center. He specified that pavilion hospitals constructed under his charge—at Chattanooga, Kingston (Tennessee), and elsewhere—should contain only two rows of bunks and incorporate additional vents to supplement the ward's windows to ensure an adequate flow of fresh air. Moore thought the topic of military-hospital planning important enough to appoint a panel of surgeons to report on their ideal placement, construction, and design.[20]

Designating General Hospitals by State

The Confederate Congress was slow to take decisive action regarding general hospitals. The January 1862 committee report from the Provisional Congress, which had praised state hospitals, recommended that more hospital space be provided and that the facilities needed more surgeons and assistants as well as a corps of competent and caring nurses. In April a House committee of the now bicameral Congress reported that government hospitals in and around Richmond, with a capacity of 5,000–6,000 patients, lagged somewhat behind state hospitals in the cleanliness of bedding and availability of "delicacies," but the care provided in them would be "amply sufficient" if existing regulations were properly enforced. Although Richmond's ability to accommodate patients had expanded since the First Battle of Manassas, it still proved woefully inadequate for casualties associated with the 1862 Peninsular Campaign, particularly those from the Battle of Seven Pines and the Seven Days' Battles.[21]

In the wake of those engagements, legislators in both houses asserted that many sick and wounded soldiers had been abused or neglected by hospital surgeons. Congressman James Farrow of South Carolina opined that most of the hardship suffered by patients stemmed from "mixing up soldiers from all portions of the Confederacy, in the same hospital, and scattering men from the same neighborhood and regiment throughout all the forty or fifty different hospitals in and around [Richmond]." He proposed drafting a bill requiring soldier-patients of each state "to be collected together, or as nearly adjacent to each other as possible." The legislator anticipated that the Medical Department would consider such a requirement impracticable, but if Congress would "will that this thing shall be done . . . then it will be practicable enough." Some objections, predicted Farrow, would arise from "incompetent and unfaithful surgeons" who feared that capable civilian assistants and nurses flocking to their state hospitals to lend their assistance would disrupt the "ease and comfort" of those medical officers and "bear testimony to derelictions of duty." Judah P. Benjamin, while secretary of war (September 1861–March 1862), had actually issued regulations in the fall of 1861, one section of which directed the Confederate Army of the Potomac "to keep the men of the same regiments and States together as nearly as possible" when assigning the sick to hospitals. That specification seemed not to apply to other armies and did not mention wounded soldiers. After large battles, the distribution of the wounded for care may have seemed haphazard but depended largely on the availability of transportation and of open beds, so patients from one state could be scattered among numerous hospitals despite all intentions to comply with Benjamin's directive.[22]

Rev. William A. Crocker, chaplain of the Fourteenth Virginia Infantry, found it nearly impossible to find men from his unit among Richmond's official and improvised hospitals after the Battle of Seven Pines and realized that countless other searchers were having the same difficulty. He thus obtained approval from the War Department to establish an organization to determine patients' whereabouts from lists provided by each Richmond facility housing the sick and wounded and to make the information available to anyone on request. On being asked by Crocker for his cooperation, Surgeon General Moore exclaimed, "Utopian, utopian!" and explained the practical difficulties of collecting the desired information. He finally ended up supporting the aims of the Army Intelligence Office, at it came to be called, and its value was such that similar services were later proposed for the Army of Tennessee—where the function was already being performed—and ordered in the Trans-Mississippi Department. The surgeon general no doubt appreciated the difficulties arising from the scattering of patients with little or no regard to their home state, but it is unclear whether he believed there was a workable solution.[23]

A Senate committee reported in late September 1862 that complaints about army hospitals, although well founded, were "in no manner attributable to the inattention or neglect of the surgeons in charge" and that the Medical Department had no control over the underlying causes of the problems. That report led to approval of legislation on September 27 that made significant changes to the operation of general hospitals; the act was put into effect via AIGO general orders on November 25. In recognition of superior conditions and survival when women were employed in hospitals, the law allowed for each hospital to employ two chief matrons, two assistant matrons, two ward matrons, ward masters, and male or female nurses and cooks. To promote patient satisfaction, account for states' rights sentiments, encourage donations from states, and facilitate the finding of individual patients, the act specified that hospitals be "known and numbered as hospitals of a particular State" and that, when practicable, patients be sent to hospitals, including state and private facilities, representing their state. Assigning patients this way was also intended to facilitate the proper expenditure of and Confederate reimbursement for funds and supplies furnished by individual states for the care of their soldiers.[24]

Consolidation of Confederate Governmental Control

By November 1862, other additional large pavilion hospitals—Winder and Howard's Grove—had opened to treat casualties sent to Richmond, and the Medical Department began to designate individual hospitals and the separate divisions of the pavilion complexes, including Chimborazo Hospital, for the various Confederate states. Assignment of patients to hospitals on the basis of state may have been facilitated by the designation of Richmond's General Hospital no. 9 (formerly called Seabrook's Hospital) in October 1862 as a receiving hospital, where sick and wounded soldiers arriving in Richmond were gathered before being transferred to other facilities. The availability of the large complexes allowed the government to begin consolidating its control of general hospitals by closing or assuming the management of private and state hospitals. Between September 1862 and March 1864, 35 Richmond hospitals were closed, starting with buildings that had only recently been appropriated to help manage the deluge of patients earlier in 1862. Next came privately operated hospitals and hospitals that had originally been established by states, although the control of some had in the meantime been assumed by the government.[25]

Surgeon General Moore was wary about being too quick to close private hospitals run by women. When William A. Carrington, then acting medical director for the Department of North Carolina and Southern Virginia, which included Richmond, suggested closing private hospitals, Moore recommended that "the better plan appears to be to let these private hospitals alone for the present. As the ladies are very desirous of attending to sick soldiers, they should be gratified." Carrington took the advice to heart, for just two weeks later, he warned Surgeon Peter E. Hines, in charge of hospitals at Petersburg, to alert the women associated with a hospital there before closing it temporarily. "[The ladies] must be consulted in regard to its permanent closure. This being a popular government we cannot disregard so important a power." He agreed not to close Robertson Hospital, a highly regarded private facility in Richmond operated by Sallie Tompkins, if strict conditions were met. "It has been very unpleasant and mortifying to me to oppose the wishes of ladies," Carrington wrote Tompkins, "especially in a matter that belongs to the public service only and should not be made personal."[26]

Representatives of at least two states believed that Moore's actions regarding their hospitals were unfair. North Carolina surgeon general Edward Warren claimed that Moore reneged on an agreement to transfer control of hospitals in Petersburg and Raleigh back to North Carolina after the state had turned them over to the Confederate government. According to North Carolinian Thomas Fanning Wood, private citizens from his state were so generous in their contributions that the storerooms of Moore Hospital in Richmond, regarded as that state's facility, were "filled with every delicacy." The SGO, said Wood, demanded that those goods be shared with other hospitals, an act that "created an angry controversy that was for a long time kept up." He also described a disagreement with Moore "in regard to the equality of State and Confederate States commissions [for surgeons]," a situation that "engendered a strife which was exhibited on sundry occasions as the war progressed." Murdoch John McSween, a North Carolina soldier who contributed his observations to the *Fayetteville Observer* under the pseudonym "Long Grabs," reported in November 1862, "The C. S. Surgeon General, I am informed, dislikes the action of Congress in classifying Hospitals according to States." In 1863 another North Carolina newspaper declared, "This man Moore, we understand, entertains a peculiar dislike for North Carolina." Judge A. F. Hopkins, whose wife was largely responsible for establishing Richmond's Alabama hospitals, believed that Surgeon General Moore had always disliked those establishments and guaranteed their demise by sending sick and wounded Alabama soldiers to other facilities.[27]

In response to "the excellent health of the soldiers of the Army of Northern Virginia" during late 1863 and early 1864, Moore had additional hospitals closed, some just temporarily in case of later need. General Lee suggested that even more be shuttered so that the soldiers detailed to work in them might be returned to the field. Moore objected strenuously, raising two important points. First, the detailed soldiers were not able-bodied, as General Lee apparently believed, and would thus not be useful in the field. Second, said Moore: "If there should be a deficiency of hospital accommodation for the sick and wounded of our armies on whom will the odium fall? Not, surely, on General Lee, but on the chief of the medical department. The want of hospitals was terribly felt in 1861, and I dare not assume the responsibility of having such scenes acted over again. Whenever it is to the interest of the service to close hospitals it has been done. At present it is not deemed advisable to discontinue any more."[28]

The occupancy of Virginia hospitals, in fact, could fluctuate widely. In April 1864, for example, 5,164 patients remained in Richmond-area hospitals, but that number jumped to 19,495 the next month, probably as a result of the Overland Campaign. Surgeon Carrington, by then medical director of Virginia hospitals, feared a severe shortage of hospital surgeons and urged Moore to temporarily relieve one medical officer from each examining board in the South that was evaluating the fitness of conscripts; those surgeons would report to Carrington for assignment. He and Moore then discussed hospital duty for surgeons who were on boards that were examining candidates to become medical officers. Those men were generally regarded as highly competent, and Carrington recommended that they "be assigned to the sole care of from 50 to 70 patients in some Hos. [hospitals] that most require skillful attention and operative interference." One drawback, he admitted, would be that "those now on duty will with reluctance and mortification see the minor duties for their patients left for them to perform and the capital operations [amputations, for example] to which attach more éclat left for them [the newly reassigned surgeons] to perform unless . . . acknowledged reputation for superior judgement and skill in operative surgery has been acquired."[29]

Why Congress believed that the numbering of general hospitals had to be legislated, as was done in the act of September 27, 1862, is unclear. For Richmond hospitals, numbering actually started on August 1, 1862, by order—probably at Moore's direction—of Surgeon Sorrel, Richmond's inspector of hospitals. At least one member of the House of Representatives took a particular interest in ensuring that Richmond's hospitals were indeed apportioned by state. Congressman William N. H. Smith of North Carolina, in April 1863 and February 1864, introduced resolutions calling on President Davis to show whether the numbering and apportionment had occurred as mandated—he seemed interested only in Richmond-area hospitals and in no other specifications of the act—and whether hospitals assigned to receive a certain state's soldiers also had surgeons from the same state. (Having hospitals for certain states staffed by surgeons from those states was not a requirement of the 1862 act.) Perhaps Smith believed that Moore's actions had to be examined to ensure that the surgeon general's purported prejudices against North Carolina—and possibly other states—were not keeping him from carrying out the conditions of the legislation.[30]

In response to the resolutions, Medical Director Carrington told Moore that the apportionment had occurred for Richmond hospitals but was impracticable for hospitals outside of the city because it would necessitate transferring thousands of patients. The original assignment of patients to hospitals took into account the availability of beds and ability of the Quartermaster and Subsistence Departments to supply the various facilities. "In military matters," said Carrington, "we have not the choice of circumstances, and what is desirable must yield to what is expedient and necessary." Furthermore, he noted, the advantages of the apportionment were balanced by "a considerable increase in expense." In addition, "Further steps have been taken to carry out the spirit of the act by registering each man entering any hospl. in the Dept., and any changes in his condition or location." Thus, by making available in his office information on the disposition of hospital patients, Carrington was duplicating the work of the Army Intelligence Office and acknowledging that making patients easier to find was an important motive behind the state apportionment of hospitals. Surgeons whom he consulted agreed that medical officers should be assigned where they could best serve the country, not according to their home state. Moore reported to President Davis in 1864 that about half of the hospital surgeons in Richmond were from the state for which their hospital was designated and that this pattern generally held for hospitals throughout the Confederacy. One factor that may have worked against such assignments was Moore's ordering medical directors to avoid assigning surgeons "to the charge of hospitals in their own place of residence." He had learned that surgeons assigned to a hometown hospital were reluctant to abandon or vacate their facility when the need arose and often neglected their patients while attending to their own private affairs.[31]

In March 1863 the Senate debated a bill (S. 7), which called for army hospitals to be "under strict and absolute military control" (rather than under the control of surgeons) and for patients to be under guard during transit from camp to hospital and from hospital to camp. An amendment to the bill called for convalescent soldiers, if deemed able by their surgeons, to undergo drill to help maintain military discipline and restore fitness for a return to active duty. Senator Louis T. Wigfall of South Carolina asserted that physicians were in the army for their professional abilities, should not hold command themselves, and should—along with other "quasi-military officers, such as commissaries and quartermasters"—be commanded by officers of the line. Guards were needed, he said, to "prevent convalescents from straggling off and poisoning themselves at whiskey shops." Opponents of the bill feared that surgeons, with the assimilated rank of major, would feel degraded if commanded by lieutenants or captains and that hospitals would effectively be turned into prisons. Senator James L. Orr, also of South Carolina, argued that the current hospital system, which had been skillfully refined by the surgeon general, would be upset by placing the facilities under military control, they already being subject to too much interference. After much discussion—and no doubt to the relief of Surgeon General Moore—the bill was rejected.[32]

Specialty Wards and Hospitals

One factor that may have complicated assigning patients to state hospitals was the advent of specialty hospitals. Those with dangerous and highly contagious diseases, such as smallpox, were typically relegated to a special ward of a general hospital or sent to a separate facility. Results of this practice were not always positive. Sending about three hundred patients with hospital gangrene to the Empire Hospital at Vineville, Georgia, was cited by Surgeon Joseph Jones as an example of a "doubtful if not dangerous and disastrous policy." Wounded men there who did not already have hospital gangrene, said Jones, always contracted it, and those convalescing from the disease often reacquired it and died. Surgeon General Moore ordered that hospitals set aside separate wards for convalescent patients and those with contagious diseases, particularly recognizing smallpox as requiring isolation. Thus, medical directors of hospitals likely needed no special approval from him to establish separate smallpox hospitals; the same probably held true for gangrene units.[33]

Confederate surgeons also established specialty hospitals for patients with other disorders. Doing so brought those with particular diagnoses together with physicians who were experienced or skilled at treating the maladies. Specialty hospitals might also facilitate the consistent gathering of statistics—a special interest of the surgeon general's—and provide settings for rudimentary medical research. Thus, the Army of Tennessee sent soldiers with venereal diseases—known to be sexually transmitted and not requiring isolation—to a hospital in Kingston, Georgia. The same army had, also in Georgia, at least one hospital for "unhealed wounds and deformities" at Cuthbert and an ophthalmic hospital that moved from Athens to Forsyth to Americus. In Virginia Medical Director Carrington ordered in 1864 that Richmond's St.

Francis de Sales Hospital should receive cases of amputation or resection (surgical removal of the damaged part of a limb bone) only. In February 1865 he directed the opening of an orthopedic facility in Richmond "for the exclusive treatment of cases of old injuries & deformities from gun shot wounds."[34]

In June 1864 Carrington informed Surgeon General Moore of the presence of patients "in various stages of mania and dementia" in Virginia's military hospitals. Although such cases were "generally given up to friends to be cared for at home or at state hosp. asylums," the state facilities were full, and many could not be sent home. Consequently, he asked Moore to establish a hospital "for cases of lunacy and dementia" in North Carolina or at some central location. It is unclear whether Carrington's request was approved, but in March 1865 he ordered the surgeon in charge of Richmond's Louisiana Hospital to prepare accommodations for twelve to fifteen "soldiers of unsound mind." Although that facility usually accepted patients from Louisiana, Surgeon General Moore had believed that only a small area would be needed for patients with mental illness and that their presence would not interfere with the building's use as a state hospital. Carrington planned to ask medical officers at Staunton, Virginia, to help secure the services of "several experienced nurses from the State Lunatic Asylum." The surgeon general knew of, or at least approved, the hospitals for the mentally ill.[35]

Moore realized the importance of dental care as well and supported a petition to exempt dentists with ten years of practice experience from conscription so that they could serve their communities. Dentist W. Leigh Burton estimated in January 1864 that there were only 250–300 dentists in areas of the Confederacy not controlled by Union forces. By late February 1864 he had been appointed as a hospital steward. Surgeons in Richmond hospitals were to gather those in need of dental operations so that Burton could visit at a convenient time and perform the necessary procedures. Moore ordered that Burton be supplied with an ambulance to save time and help transport his instruments. In November 1864 Surgeon Carrington announced that dental operations would be performed in general hospitals by "officers, soldiers or conscripts assigned to those duties who are dentists by profession."[36]

In early 1865 Moore ordered medical directors of hospitals to select a well-lighted ward in one of their facilities for patients with fractured jaws to be fitted with an apparatus called an interdental splint, designed by a civilian dentist named James Baxter Bean. Surgeon Stout had met Bean in Atlanta, where the dentist offered to treat Confederate soldiers free of charge. Stout was impressed with the effectiveness of Bean's splint and subsequently ordered that patients with jaw fractures be sent to Atlanta's Medical College Hospital, where Bean could treat them. Surgeon Edward N. Covey, who was inspecting area hospitals, learned of his success and evidently informed the surgeon general, who asked Bean to visit Richmond to demonstrate the device. The result was Moore's order as described above. Medical Director Carrington selected a ward in Richmond's General Hospital No. 9 for treatment with the splint and ordered surgeons in Richmond and Petersburg to send eligible patients.[37]

Carrington also ordered that special wards at Howard's Grove, Winder, Jackson, and Chimborazo Hospitals be set aside for investigating the effects of various indigenous remedies for malaria. Each research area was to be under the command of one medical officer, and the medications were to be given singly so that their effects could be determined. Since Moore had a special interest in indigenous remedies, there is little doubt that Carrington's order was issued under the surgeon general's direction.[38]

A May 1, 1863, amendment to the act of September 27, 1862, directed the surgeon general to establish way (or wayside) hospitals at convenient points along railroads to house and feed sick and disabled soldiers traveling home on furlough or who had been honorably discharged from the army. These were to be operated in the same manner as general hospitals. This was accomplished, in part, by assuming control of some of the larger preexisting way hospitals earlier established by local women's groups.[39]

Moore's Overall Influence on General Hospitals

Listings in the fall of 1864 showed a large collection of Confederate "principal hospitals" east of the Mississippi. Nineteen were clearly identified as way hospitals, and the balance—presumably general hospitals—numbered forty-nine in Georgia, thirty-six in Virginia, nineteen in Alabama, fourteen in North Carolina, nine in South Carolina, three in Florida, and two each in Mississippi and Tennessee. It is difficult to generalize about the extent to which Moore personally controlled major decisions about general hospitals in the Confederacy. During the first half of the war, they were within the purview of medical directors of military commands, and during the latter half, medical directors of hospitals assumed that responsibility. Both types of medical director reported to Moore, but the point at which their actions were subject to his approval is unclear. Because of delays in communication and Moore's unfamiliarity with the exact circumstances at sites far removed from Richmond, the independence of medical directors probably increased with their distance from the capital. Although he had placed Sorrel in charge of all general hospitals east of the Mississippi, the surgeon general had good reason to take more personal responsibility for hospitals in and about Richmond. The city was, after all, the Confederacy's major medical center, and its facilities were readily available for criticism by politicians, newspaper correspondents, and others. Although few surviving orders from the SGO bear a signature other than Moore's, the vastness of the surgeon general's responsibilities suggests that many decisions regarding general hospitals were formulated by his trusted staff but enacted under his signature.[40]

Moore's struggles to establish a functional general-hospital system was generally supported by legislation aimed at supplying adequate funds and personnel, but President Davis's approval of bills was far from automatic. Beside the constant shortages of supplies and manpower, Moore's challenges included dealing with individuals and groups who placed the interests of their state over those of the central government, charitable groups and private citizens who wished to operate hospitals on their own terms, and legislators who believed they knew more about hospital management than he did. Within the army itself, he had to work with elements that were unable or uncooperative, such as the Quartermaster and Subsistence Departments, or had competing interests, such as commanders like General Lee, who sought hospital workers to join their fighting ranks. The ability of the general-hospital system to function at all in spite of such hindrances demonstrates the skills of the surgeon general and the dedication of his medical officers.[41]

10. ❖ Prison Hospitals

Among Surgeon General Moore's responsibilities was the operation of hospitals for Union prisoners of war (POWs). After the war he was portrayed as a villain for his alleged part in the maltreatment of POWs, especially those confined at the notorious Andersonville Prison in Georgia. Existing documents show some of his actions regarding POWs but are much less helpful in providing a complete view of his beliefs and motives.

How Moore oversaw prison hospitals was heavily influenced by how prisons themselves were operated. The Confederate government struggled throughout the war with a muddled command structure for confining and caring for POWs. Custody and sustenance of POWs were officially the responsibility of the quartermaster general under instructions of the secretary of war. Responsibility for providing them rations was unofficially transferred from the quartermaster general to the commissary general of subsistence in August 1863, a change formalized in February 1864. Prison hospitals sometimes constituted separate buildings, such as factories and warehouses, but might also occupy a particular section of a prison building or camp. Where these facilities were located and how much space they occupied were determined primarily by the prison commandant if onsite or by another officer if outside the prison compound.[1]

That other officer was often Brigadier General John H. Winder, inspector general of the military camps around Richmond starting in June 1861. Winder, the de facto commander of prisons in Richmond and in much of the South, lacked sufficient official command authority throughout most of the war. That changed somewhat after he was named commander of the post at Andersonville in June 1864. The next month he was given command of military prisons in Georgia and Alabama and directed to communicate with and receive orders from Adjutant and Inspector General Cooper. In November 1864 Winder was appointed commissary general of prisoners and given formal control of prisons east of the Mississippi River. Regardless of his title, the most important decisions about POWs were made by Winder's superiors—in particular, the secretary of war and General Cooper.[2]

126

As if to verify that confusion existed about the operation of prison hospitals, the AIGO decreed in late 1863—at Moore's urging—that such facilities were "on the same footing as other C.S. hospitals in all respects" and would be managed accordingly. Thus, surgeons assigned to prison hospitals would report to their respective medical director of hospitals, who was responsible to the surgeon general. But Surgeon William A. Carrington, medical director of Virginia hospitals, stated on July 12, 1864, that prison hospitals under his control and supervision were "governed by military law through the military authorities." He was referring to Winder, for in March 1863 the AIGO had clouded matters by naming him as commander of general hospitals—presumably including prison hospitals—in Richmond.[3]

In January 1865, when Winder was commanding "all officers and men serving with the different prisons east of the Mississippi River," he informed Surgeon General Moore that he had appointed Surgeon Isaiah H. White, formerly chief surgeon at Andersonville, as chief medical officer of prisons. "The interest of the prisons being somewhat at variance with the Confederate hospitals," said Winder, "great difficulty is sometimes experienced in obtaining the necessary supplies for the comfort of the sick of this command." Another complication, he noted, was that, because prisons had to relocate frequently, it was necessary to transfer their medical officers beyond the limits of their home military department. Winder wished surgeons serving in prison hospitals to report to Surgeon White rather than to medical directors of hospitals and to have White report directly to Moore.[4]

In characterizing how POWs were managed by both the South and the North, it is useful to divide the war roughly into three phases. The first, which lasted from the commencement of hostilities until late July 1862, was characterized by massive prison overcrowding as both sides dealt with an unanticipated scale and duration of war. The second, starting in July 1862 and lasting about a year, encompassed a cartel that allowed the regular exchange of numerous Union and Confederate POWs and generally eased overcrowding in prisons outside of Richmond. The third phase, starting in mid-1863, saw the cartel fall apart, prison populations swell, and prison conditions deteriorate. In Richmond, independent of the cartel, conditions in prison hospitals worsened with influxes of large numbers of wounded Confederate and Union soldiers, as occurred after battles near the Confederate capital. The city's prison population also grew as captives were gathered there in preparation for exchange. Explaining the changing conditions and comparing how the Confederacy and Union treated POWs are beyond the scope of this study, yet the actions of Surgeon General Moore and other Confederate officials must be considered in the context of the aforementioned phases and influences. This discussion focuses on the two most troublesome phases, those that occurred early and late in the war.[5]

Early War: Overcrowding

Prison overcrowding was an early problem. On August 1, 1861, shortly after the First Battle of Manassas and just two days after being appointed acting surgeon general, Moore reported to Secretary of War Walker that the Richmond buildings housing Union POWs already were overcrowded and not properly policed. He feared "that a pestilence may make its appearance, and if it should the city would be the sufferer." Although Moore did not, in that communication, express direct concern for the prisoners' well-being, he may have calculated that a threat to Richmond's populace would prompt quick corrective action. The surgeon general reported that he had asked Brigadier General Winder to ensure that cleanliness was attended to and advised Walker that another prison building was needed. Moore, ever the stickler for military protocol, would probably not have gone over Winder's head to Walker unless he had been dissatisfied by his interaction with the general.[6]

On being directed by Walker to remedy the situation, Winder stated that Moore's complaints were premature. The overcrowding, he insisted, had occurred entirely because one of the prison buildings had been quickly vacated, at Moore's request, for use as a hospital for Confederate soldiers. Since Winder did not immediately have space for the displaced prisoners elsewhere, he had squeezed them into other structures already housing POWs. The lack of cleanliness resulted from this overcrowding, which again stemmed from Moore's request. The accuracy of Winder's explanation is debatable, for it required Moore to have asked him to empty one prison building, allowed time for that to happen, and then visited the newly overcrowded buildings, all within two days of becoming acting surgeon general. Throughout the war, Winder tended to acknowledge poor conditions in prisons but to consistently blame factors supposedly beyond his control. Andersonville historian Ovid Futch characterized the general as disputatious when dealing with colleagues, and biographer Arch Blakey called him abrupt, short tempered, and—during late stages of the war—"more hardened to the suffering of his captives." Yet Winder was untiring in his efforts to improve conditions for POWs, but his pleas often went unanswered by his superiors.[7]

In June 1862 Colonel Stephen A. Dodge, a wounded Union officer being treated in a Richmond hospital, begged Secretary of War Randolph to authorize his parole and send him home for fear he would contract erysipelas (now known to be a streptococcal skin infection) and die. Randolph told the surgeon general that he wished Dodge transferred to another hospital if appropriate, and Moore accompanied Surgeon Francis Sorrel, inspector of hospitals, to examine the patient. Although erysipelas had indeed appeared in some patients, Dodge's wound was found "in a healthy condition." Whether to parole him was not Moore's decision, and the officer declined a transfer if he could not be paroled. Nevertheless, Moore's personal participation in this matter seems to indicate that he did not lack concern for prisoners' welfare. Confederate officials cared enough about controlling contagion that in mid-1862 they established a separate hospital for the isolation and treatment of Union POWs with hospital gangrene, a virulent necrotizing infection.[8]

Various medical officers were vocal about what they perceived as mistreatment of POWs. Surgeon Carrington, then inspector of hospitals, reported on conditions in Richmond's prison hospitals in October 1862. He found that the Castle Thunder hospital, where Confederate stragglers and alleged deserters were confined, was overcrowded and lacked a bathroom, linen room, and hospital clothing. "The beds & bedding were filthy," said Carrington, "& the clothing and persons of the patients in the same condition." The two buildings containing hospitals for Union POWs lacked bathrooms, and their privies were poorly constructed and in poor condition. There, too, the bedding, floors, and patients themselves were "filthy & disgusting" and general order was lacking, but—unlike later in the war—at least the food was well prepared and available in adequate amounts. All hospitals included in Carrington's reports were attended by contract surgeons. The inspector did not indicate that POWs were more poorly treated than the Confederate prisoners at Castle Thunder and did not mention overcrowding. "The inmates of these Hospls are our disarmed & frequently disabled enemies," wrote Carrington. "A respect for the opinion of foreign nations, humanity, chivalry & Christianity & even policy would make it eminently desirable" to make the changes he recommended. Some of Carrington's suggested remedies, such as assigning Confederate surgeons to take charge of the facilities and providing a sufficient number of hospital attendants, could—if the personnel were available—be enacted by the surgeon general. But Moore had little or no authority regarding the selection of spaces allowed for prison hospitals and had to depend on the secretary of war, the Quartermaster Department, and Brigadier General Winder to make major decisions about the facilities.[9]

Late War: Deterioration

In July 1863, as the exchange cartel was breaking down, Surgeon General Moore wrote to Secretary of War Seddon about conditions described to him by a Confederate soldier recently released from the Union prison at Fort Delaware. The high death rate among the inmates there, said Moore, was attributable to their being kept in its "overcrowded and pestilential cells and to their being subjected to the use of unwholesome food and bad water." He called the prisoners' treatment a "seemingly unworthy attempt to subdue or destroy our soldiers by pestilence and disease" and "unmerciful and unjust conduct" by the US government. Humane treatment and efforts to prevent the spread of disease were beneficial for captives and captors alike, he asserted, repeating the reasoning he used when arguing for more room for POWs in Richmond. "And how much more," added Moore, "does the propriety of this course become evident on appeal to the code of civilization and to the dictates of Christianity." In referring to ethical conduct, he echoed the sentiments expressed several months earlier when Surgeon Carrington recommended better treatment of POWs. Whether Moore's indignity at the treatment of Confederate POWs colored his views about how Union captives should be handled remains uncertain.[10]

Moore's reaction to the report about Fort Delaware coincided with decisions that would result in new levels of suffering by Union POWs. Officials had been reluctant to expand or improve facilities for captives during the cartel because prisons were being emptied. Even as the system became inoperative, inattention to facilities continued because exchange was expected to resume. Because that did not occur, existing prisons and their hospitals became increasingly crowded, and new, ill-prepared facilities filled quickly. Prison commandants reported that they could not accommodate additional inmates, yet officials continued issuing orders to send them more POWs while declining to provide adequate rations and other supplies. An early act of the Provisional Congress had specified that rations given to POWs should "be the same in quantity and quality as those furnished to enlisted men in the army of the Confederacy." But in August 1863 Commissary General Lucius B. Northrop and the quartermaster general agreed, with the approval of Secretary of War Seddon, that if food became scarce enough to differentiate between Confederate soldiers at stationary posts and those in the field, troops in the field—because they were more active—would be favored over those at posts as well as over POWS. Should provisions became even scarcer, Confederate soldiers would be favored over Union captives in the distribution of meat. Northrop had chronic difficulty procuring enough food for the army and, according to War Department clerk John B. Jones, wanted to remove meat from POW rations altogether and substitute "oat gruel, corn-meal gruel, and pea soup, soft hominy, and bread." Northrop's motive, said Jones, was retaliation for the Union's poor treatment of Confederate POWs and for Federal soldiers' destruction of the South's ability to raise and harvest crops.[11]

Medical officers began to suspect a deliberate intent behind the neglect of POWs. Surgeon Carrington had repeatedly informed Brigadier General Winder and Surgeon General Moore of overcrowding and high death rates in Richmond's prison hospitals. In March 1864 he reported that Moore had, in a private interview, referred to the matter as "one of international policy and military control." Inspections of Richmond prisons and hospitals conducted by a congressional committee and by Confederate officers, themselves former POWs, had "reported favorably and approvingly" in what Carrington clearly saw as a purposeful attempt to conceal the truth. "At this time," he stated, "I adopted the conviction that the existing state of things was known and approved by the [War] Department for the purposes of diplomatic policy, or forced upon them by the stern necessities of the occasion." Carrington declared himself not responsible for the poor conditions: "I did all I could by proper supply of officers and directions to them to avoid imputation that the medical department could legitimately be considered as compromised by or responsible for the existing regulations adopted by the necessities of military law." Winder acknowledged that conditions in Richmond prisons were less than "most conducive to their [POWs'] health and comfort" but suggested that "mortality is incident to prison life, and cannot reasonably be attributed to the want of space in the hospitals."[12]

Surgeon Tobias G. Richardson inspected Richmond's prison hospitals on orders from General Bragg, military advisor to President Davis. In an April 1864 letter to Bragg, the surgeon disagreed with Winder's dismissal of overcrowding as a critical problem and blamed the "fearful mortality" in prison hospitals on that and filthy conditions. He also referred to Surgeon Carrington's impression that "the refusal of proper accommodations to the sick Federal prisoners was one of State policy," adding that Winder seemed "to some extent influenced by a similar impression."[13]

Indeed, historian Charles W. Sanders Jr. has argued that the horrendous conditions in prisons and their hospitals were known by senior Confederate officials, including President Davis, and that Secretary of War Seddon and

Adjutant and Inspector General Cooper deliberately issued orders that worsened overcrowding. When deciding how resources should be allotted between Confederate troops and POWs, they chose to seriously shortchange the latter. Possibly contributing to those decisions were callousness—developed as the war became more brutal—a desire to retaliate for Union mistreatment of Confederate captives, and public pressure to devote scarce resources to Southern citizenry rather than to POWs. Attempts to treat prisoners humanely were no doubt hampered by the South's widespread shortages of food and other supplies, unreliable transportation networks, and poor prison management, but the efforts were nevertheless considered to be of low importance relative to the government's other worries. That ranking of priorities led to the inevitable consequences of malnutrition, rampant disease, and death among POWs.[14]

The Wirz Trial

Whether Surgeon General Moore participated in setting those priorities, agreed with them, or had the power to mitigate them is difficult to determine from existing records. His alleged involvement in the mistreatment of POWs arose in the military trial of Henry Wirz, former commander of the prison stockade at Andersonville. The outrage in the North that followed the assassination of President Lincoln and the thirst for retribution for the Confederacy's mistreatment of Union POWs made Wirz's conviction and execution foregone conclusions. His trial—called a "legal lynching" by historian Ovid Futch—was patently unfair and sought to brand high-ranking Confederate officials as inhumane. Thus, claims made against Moore by the trial's prosecutor must be viewed with caution.[15]

Two charges were filed against Wirz when trial proceedings began in August 1865. The first was for conspiracy "to injure the health and destroy the lives" of Union POWs. In its original form, the charge named as coconspirators Robert E. Lee, Seddon, Winder (who had died in February 1865), Northrop (former commissary general of subsistence), former Andersonville surgeons Isaiah H. White and R. Randolph Stevenson, former surgeon general Moore, two additional named individuals, and "others unknown." The second charge was murder, with thirteen specifications involving unnamed POWs. The names of Lee, Seddon, Northrop, and Moore were removed from the conspiracy charge at the insistence of US secretary of war Edwin M. Stanton, an alteration that baffled Judge Advocate Norton P. Chipman. Among the former Confederate officials subpoenaed for the defense were Lee, Seddon, and Moore; Moore actually traveled to Washington, DC, to appear in court. Chipman, however, revoked the subpoenas on the grounds that those individuals were implicated in the charges against Wirz and were therefore legally incompetent to testify for the defense until they were acquitted in court or officially pardoned; they could, however, testify for the prosecution (but none did).[16]

In October Wirz was found guilty of conspiracy and of most of the specifications of murder and sentenced to death; he was hanged the next month. In the official findings the conspiracy charge was modified "to conform with the facts" presented at the trial: Davis, Seddon, and Moore, but not Lee or Northrop, were added as coconspirators. It is curious that Cooper, former adjutant and inspector general, was not included in any version of the conspiracy charge. The verdict, said Chipman, although "not tantamount to the conviction of the alleged conspirators [including Moore], other than Wirz," was "the equivalent of an indictment found against them for complicity in this wholesale and needless mortality." With Wirz's execution, he recalled, "the secondary, but really most important, result of the trial [the proof of conspiracy at the highest levels of the Confederate government], passed out of mind, or was displaced by the rapidly recurring political movements of that eventful period." Chipman was evidently referring to President Andrew Johnson becoming lenient toward former Confederate leaders after his initial determination to see them punished. Of Wirz's alleged coconspirators, only former soldier James W. Duncan, employed in the commissary at Andersonville, was tried; he was convicted of manslaughter. The only other former Confederate tried for war crimes—John H. Gee, who had commanded the prison at Salisbury, North Carolina—was acquitted.[17]

Moore's inclusion as a coconspirator resulted largely from his directing Surgeon Joseph Jones to visit Andersonville to research the causes of sickness and death among the POWs there. Jones, who specialized in gathering and interpreting scientific data, became aware of the high mortality rates at Andersonville and obtained the surgeon general's permission to investigate personally. In ordering Andersonville surgeon White to accommodate Jones, Moore indicated that the efforts were "for the benefit of the medical department of the Confederate armies." During the trial, Chipman portrayed White as cruel and incompetent and blasted Moore not only for keeping him in place but also for sending an "eminent medical gentleman" (Jones) to conduct research rather than to help care for patients. To the coldblooded Moore, he claimed, Andersonville "was a mere dissecting room, a clinic institute to be made tributary to the medical department of the Confederate armies." It was difficult, Chipman said, "to conceive with what devilish malice, or criminal devotion to his profession, or reckless disregard of the high duties imposed upon him," Moore could instruct Surgeon Jones to study the situation at Andersonville. To illustrate the former surgeon general's alleged callousness, the prosecutor cited his "flippant" endorsement on Surgeon White's report that he was short of medical supplies and that medical officers were needed to replace departing contract surgeons. "Not having supplies," read Moore's endorsement, "is his [White's] own fault; he should have anticipated the wants of the sick by timely requisitions. . . . It is impossible to order medical officers in place of the contract physicians. They are not to be had at present." In fact, there seems to have been nothing untrue in Moore's remark, and he was terse by nature, especially in endorsements.[18]

Surgeon Jones prepared a lengthy report, in which he described in great detail the horrid conditions at Andersonville, presented statistics on the prevalence of disease and causes of death, and offered suggestions for improving the health of the inmates. After leaving Andersonville, he visited general hospitals in Macon, Vineville, and Columbus, Georgia, to similarly study the illnesses afflicting Confederate soldiers. The latter visits were in accordance with the wishes of Surgeon General Moore, expressed in a circular issued on the same day (August 6, 1864) as the order for Surgeon White to cooperate with Jones. Because of Federal military advances and transportation difficulties in Georgia in late 1864, the investigator never sent his Andersonville report to Moore. Chipman somehow learned of the report and ordered Jones in September 1865 to come to Washington, DC, to testify at the Wirz trial and to bring all documents in his possession pertaining to Andersonville. Jones was mortified. His report "was prepared solely for the eye of the Surgeon-General of the Confederate States Army," and its frankness, he feared, "would only engender angry feelings, and place weapons in the hands of the victors."[19]

Decades after the war, Francis Sorrel, formerly of the Confederate SGO, recalled that Jones, while at Andersonville, had been "engaged in some new and experimental processes" related to hospital gangrene, which was rampant at the prison camp and problematic at general hospitals. His reports on the topic had been filed in the SGO. After appearing at the Wirz trial, Jones visited Sorrel in a panic, fearing that, should those reports surface, he too "might be implicated in the charge of cruelty to Federal prisoners in view of these experiments." Sorrel calmed Jones by informing him that the dispatches had been destroyed in the fire that swept Richmond in April 1865. "There was nothing in them, however," he recalled, "under a fair professional inter-pretation, to incriminate him." Nevertheless, Jones's Andersonville report documented conditions at the camp and was especially devastating because it presented the findings of an objective and observant Confederate medical officer. Chipman used its most damaging parts to help convict Wirz while omitting the descriptions of efforts taken by Confederate surgeons to ease prisoners' suffering.[20]

According to Louis Schade, defense attorney for Wirz, Chipman's re-vocation of the subpoenas for Moore and others was one illustration of the unfairness that made the trial "a wretched farce." Had Moore been allowed to testify fully, his role in the management of POWs might have been elucidated, but Schade maintained that the potential witnesses "would not have been permitted to say anything in favor of the prisoner and the cause of justice and humanity." Instead, he concluded, the witnesses "would have been subject to the overbearing insolence of the president of the Commission, General Lew Wallace, whilst at the other end of the table the Judge Advocate [Chipman], by sneering questions and insulting insinuations, would have taxed the forbear-ance of the rebels, as he politely used to denominate the Southern witnesses."[21]

Moore's Culpability

Although Surgeon General Moore's part in the mistreatment of POWs is unclear, the evidence suggests that he bore little responsibility. The decisions to overcrowd prisons and withhold adequate supplies of food and other necessities were made by Secretary of War Seddon and Adjutant and Inspector General Cooper. President Davis surely knew of the awful conditions, and he at least allowed Seddon and Cooper to control matters even if he did not openly condone the policy. Moore, previously excluded from discussions between Seddon and Cooper, was unlikely to have been involved in such decisions. He did seem aware of the unwritten policy by which POWs ranked lower than Confederate soldiers in the distribution of resources and probably recognized the futility of trying to change his superiors' minds.[22]

Whether assigning more and better surgeons to prisons and their hospitals would have benefited the health of POWs is debatable. The improvements that would have helped them the most were well known to prison commandants, were repeatedly recommended by surgeons, and would probably not have been accomplished merely because more surgeons were present. POWs suffered because the buildings or grounds that confined them were hastily prepared and became overcrowded quickly; staff never seemed to have the time, resources, or skill to organize the prisons properly. Keeping the facilities policed was difficult at best and was often neglected; consequently, the grounds became contaminated with feces, trash, and rotting food and infested with insects. Food was not supplied in adequate amounts, and the rations that were provided were unbalanced or spoiled, resulting in malnutrition, intestinal disorders, and scurvy. The cornmeal issued to POWs was unbolted—it still contained fragments of husk—and exacerbated their almost universal malady, diarrhea. Water sources were often contaminated by latrines or by receiving other waste materials. At some prisons like Andersonville, most POWs had little or no shelter and lacked adequate clothing. It would take no more than one medical officer to urge the correction of such deficiencies, after which he could only hope that the commandant agreed and could gather the resources to make the changes possible. If sick POWs were sent to the prison hospital, any recovery occurring there was most likely attributable to temporary improvements in shelter and nourishment. Patients who improved while in a prison hospital were likely to sicken again if returned to the main prison compound.[23]

Additional surgeons might have arranged for more effective isolation of patients with certain infectious diseases—hospital gangrene or smallpox, for example—but separate and additional room for patients was typically unavailable. They might also have been able to more effectively vaccinate POWs against smallpox. Jones reported, in fact, that an outbreak of smallpox at Andersonville had been arrested by vaccination. In some cases "large gangrenous ulcers" developed at vaccination sites, causing extensive tissue destruction and necessitating amputation. Some POWs (and Judge Advocate Chipman) attributed such outcomes to Confederate surgeons deliberately using poisonous materials during vaccination, but Jones believed that scurvy and overcrowding predisposed the men to develop hospital gangrene in even the smallest wound, whether it was accidental, caused by an insect bite, or resulted from vaccination.[24]

Shortages of medicines were cited as contributing to the poor health of POWs too, but the remedies available at the time would not have provided much relief. The prevailing diseases at Andersonville, according to Jones, were scurvy, diarrhea, dysentery, and hospital gangrene. Scurvy, caused by vitamin C deficiency, would not respond to medications on the army's standard supply table, none of which contained vitamin C. The medical purveyor at Macon did send small amounts of orange juice, a nonstandard item, to Andersonville, though not enough to prevent or treat scurvy in the general prison population. Dysentery and most cases of prison diarrhea were of infectious origin, acquired from the filthy surroundings or from contaminated food or water. Surgeons had no antimicrobial drugs that would prevent or cure such maladies. Opiates might temporarily control diarrhea or dull the abdominal pain of dysentery, but according to Surgeon Jones, "the frail dam was soon swept away, and the patient appeared to be but little better, if not the worse, for this merely palliative treatment." Physicians sometimes treated hospital gangrene, another infectious disease not curable with available medicines, with topical application of nitric acid and other substances—such actions may have constituted Jones's experimental treatments—but the therapies had temporary benefits at best, after which "the gangrene would frequently return with redoubled energy." Quinine, which was in short supply, could be effective against malaria, but that disease was uncommon at Andersonville. Remedies derived from indigenous Southern plants were issued by medical purveyors as substitutes for quinine and other drugs, but they were generally thought to be of little use at Andersonville and elsewhere.[25]

Robert Ould, former Confederate commissioner of exchange, wrote that "in consequence of certain information" from Surgeon General Moore, he offered in the summer of 1864 to buy medicine from US authorities for the exclusive use of POWs in Confederate prisons and even to allow US surgeons to deliver and dispense them. "To this offer," reported Ould, "I never received a reply. Incredible as this appears, it is strictly true." Infinitely more effective than available medicines would have been attention to basic principles of sanitation and the provision of adequate room, shelter, clothes, food, and water; prison surgeons, however, had little influence in such matters. As one Andersonville surgeon said, "What medicine we gave I considered thrown away, because we did not have proper diet for the patients, and consequently the medicine did no good."[26]

It is unlikely that Surgeon General Moore conspired to mistreat POWs so that he could dispatch an investigator, Surgeon Jones, to study the consequences of that mistreatment. Jones, on the same trip and in obedience to orders from Moore, researched illnesses among Confederate soldiers in general hospitals. Judge Advocate Chipman would certainly not have attached the same coldblooded motive to those visits as he did to Jones's Andersonville investigation. Moore also had a long history of encouraging surgeons to report statistics and document experiences so that the army could benefit from the collected data. The US surgeon general had encouraged Union surgeons to conduct similar documentary activities.[27]

Although Moore was never formally charged with a war crime, US officials may have considered doing so. Some former Confederates were not automatically granted amnesty after the war upon signing a loyalty oath and had to apply for pardon to the president. Such men included those "who resigned commissions in the army or navy of the United States and afterwards aided the rebellion" or who had been "engaged in any way in treating otherwise than lawfully as prisoners of war persons found in the United States service." Because Moore had served the Confederacy after resigning his commission in the US Army, he applied for pardon to President Johnson in May and June 1865. On July 3 Surgeon General Joseph K. Barnes recommended to Attorney General James Speed that Moore be pardoned. A final recommendation by Attorney General Henry Stanbery, who succeeded Speed on July 23, was delayed—seemingly by intention—until well after Wirz had been tried, convicted, and executed. Stanbery recommended again on November 30, 1866, that Moore be pardoned; it was granted the next day. (In contrast, Charles Brewer, a former US Army surgeon who became a Confederate surgeon and assisted Moore in the SGO, applied to President Johnson for pardon on May 11, 1865, and had the pardon granted after just a month, on June 12, 1865.) Whether US government officials, other than those involved in the Wirz trial, believed Moore to have been cruel to POWs is unknown, but there were few, if any, calls after the trial for Moore to be prosecuted.[28]

11. ❈ Striving for Quality in Medical Personnel

A s troops from the various Southern states were accepted into Confederate service, they were accompanied by surgeons and assistant surgeons who were elected by the soldiers or appointed by state officials but were not necessarily competent. Those medical officers at first were given commissions in the PACS by President Davis without undergoing a qualifying examination. "Little discrimination has been shown in the selection of these officers," wrote a newspaper correspondent in September 1861, "and many most inefficient Surgeons have found their way into the medical staff of the army." The problem, opined a Confederate surgeon, was that because many reputable physicians had not joined the army, the medical corps was primarily composed of relatively young men. Since the regulations required "a certain number of medical officers, they are selected from the material presented." Furthermore, he continued, "the machinations of wire pulling men" resulted in unworthy persons being appointed by the president. Such machinations, said another observer, might involve candidates for regimental colonel or major and those for surgeon supporting each other, with the result that "the appointment is given to the most successful intriguant, though he may be the poorest Surgeon." Another Confederate medical officer reported that the original surgeons of his unit were selected "by previous understanding with a wealthy and influential relative who was a large contributor to the equipment of the company."[1]

Complaints about surgeons were particularly common in the months following the First Battle of Manassas. Regimental surgeons, said one observer, were characterized by "ignorance, stupidity, and utter incompetence." One physician supposedly ventured that "the army would be better off without doctors altogether, because the good ones cannot do as much good as the incompetent do harm." These men were also criticized for their lack of experience. "Many of the Surgeons now in the service are cross-roads doctors, who never performed half a dozen surgical operations in their lives, and who know almost as little of the proper treatment of gun-shot wounds as a lawyer or a blacksmith."[2]

It would make sense, then, to examine the qualifications of men who wished to become medical officers along with those who had already been appointed. The Medical Department regulations in effect when Moore became acting surgeon general were instituted in March 1861, repeated those of the US Army, and were worded to pertain to the Confederate regular army only. They specified that the secretary of war would, from time to time, appoint boards consisting of at least three medical officers. These would examine applicants for appointment as assistant surgeon as well as assistant surgeons applying for promotion; no appointment or promotion could occur without a satisfactory examination. Applicants for assistant surgeon had to be between twenty-one and twenty-five years of age and would be scrutinized for "moral habits, professional acquirements, and physical qualifications." An assistant surgeon who had served for five years was subject to examination for promotion and would be removed from the army if he declined the examination or was found to be unqualified. An applicant who failed an examination for assistant surgeon would have a single chance, after two years, to be reexamined. It appears that no medical officers in the regular army were examined before being so appointed, and few or none of them were examined later. The fact that all had been examined by US Army medical boards earlier in their career probably sufficed.[3]

Establishment of Examining Boards

Although Medical Department regulations said nothing about examinations for medical officers in the PACS, acts of the Provisional Confederate Congress gave the president authority to appoint army officers and indicated that they must first pass "an examination satisfactory to the President, and in such manner as he may prescribe." Examination could be postponed for a year after appointment if the president deemed the delay necessary for the public good. Thus, on September 4, 1861, AIGO special orders announced the organization of two boards, each composed of three surgeons, to be governed by special instructions from Acting Surgeon General Moore. One was to hold sessions at Manassas, while the other would operate at points to be designated by Moore. Each board included a surgeon who been a medical officer in the US Army—Robert L. Brodie (resigned from Federal service in May 1861) on one, and Robert Southgate (resigned from Federal service in March 1856) on the other, assignments made, no doubt by Moore, so that the examiners would include at least one individual who had himself been examined by a medical board, albeit by a Federal one. Subsequent announcements made clear that the boards would examine medical officers and candidates hoping to become the same; that they would convene at Norfolk, Richmond, Yorktown, and Manassas, Virginia; and that they would meet "at other points farther South at a convenient time."[4]

As the war progressed, additional boards were formed. Examination locations in 1862 and 1863 included Mobile, Alabama; Pensacola and Tallahassee, Florida; Vicksburg, Mississippi; Savannah, Georgia; Goldsboro, North Carolina; Charleston, South Carolina; Nashville, Knoxville, Chattanooga, and Murfreesboro, Tennessee; and Manassas and Richmond, Virginia. Boards were also formed by January 1862 to examine applicants serving in the commands of Generals Albert Sidney Johnston and Robert E. Lee and by April for the command of Major General Sterling Price. Boards west of the Mississippi operated in the Department of Texas and West Louisiana, in Arkansas (Little Rock, Washington, and Fort Smith), and Texas (Marshall). Examinations were conducted at multiple other locations during the war.[5]

Surgeon Lafayette Guild, medical director of the Army of Northern Virginia, explained the rationale for ordering boards "to convene near or in the camp of the army." There were many surgeons who deserved promotion and wished to go to Richmond to be examined, he told Surgeon General Moore, but General Lee withheld permission to go "for the evident reason that their services cannot be spared from the regiments." Guild offered to recommend surgeons from Lee's army to constitute a board to examine its medical officers and applicants for appointment. When Moore asked for three names, Guild provided five, a number that would permit the members to attend to duties other than those pertaining to the board. (Members not associated with specific commands were relieved of other responsibilities while on board duty.) Moore agreed and appointed the five men Guild recommended.[6]

Persons desiring an appointment as surgeon or assistant surgeon were to apply to the secretary of war and include testimonials of moral character, after which they would receive an invitation to appear before a board. Surgeon Nathan Bozeman, recorder for one of the panels, reported on October 6, 1861, that instructions from the secretary of war (Judah P. Benjamin) were "peremptory to the effect that all surgeons & assistant surgeons now in the service shall be examined."[7]

Objections from Medical Officers

Whether Moore was the driving force behind starting examinations is unknown, but it seems likely that President Davis and Adjutant and Inspector

General Cooper, both accustomed to the ways of the US Army, would have supported such a move. The formation of the boards elicited some approval. In October 1861, for example, the editors of the *Southern Medical and Surgical Journal* suggested that the army adopt the standards used by the government of Ohio in examining potential medical officers: Ten years of practice should be required for appointment as surgeon and five years for assistant surgeon, with a respectable medical diploma needed in all cases.[8] The most spirited reactions were from men who had already been appointed as medical officers. On September 17, 1861, a reporter stationed at Norfolk observed: "The medical board, now in session in this place, has caused *no little excitement*. Many of the surgeons have *positively refused* to be examined. Some are very indignant. Some have resigned, and, as a general thing, *all are dissatisfied*. Something of this kind should have been established at the commencement; but to give a gentleman an appointment *and then examine* him to learn his qualifications, is a course of proceedings heretofore unheard of."[9]

The story may have been describing the medical officers of the Army of the Peninsula, who were represented by Surgeon William H. Coffin in a letter to President Davis dated October 21, 1861. Coffin asserted that having surgeons examined by other officers who had secured their commission in the same manner—by presidential appointment—was "unjust discrimination in favor of the Examiners" and was "individually degrading to each Medical Officer." Those being examined, he noted, risked being "found deficient either from improper motives or from error of judgement in the examiners." Finally, Coffin claimed that the president had no constitutional authority to remove an officer; incompetent surgeons could instead be removed by action of a court of inquiry or court-martial. Davis, in rejecting those arguments, stated that a court of inquiry was limited to examining official misconduct or moral delinquency and that professional qualification could be determined by medical men only. The authority to examine officers derived from acts signed into law on March 6.[10]

Protests arose elsewhere in the medical ranks. Surgeon James McFadden Gaston and his colleagues in Brigadier General D. R. Jones's South Carolina brigade objected to being examined on the grounds that they had already been commissioned. "Like opposition," said Gaston, "was manifested by medical officers in other commands." Since he had participated in the protest, the surgeon resigned his commission but advised his colleagues "to accept the conditions and submit to the examination." After his resignation was accepted, he reconsidered and decided "that the government had the right to require any condition for the appointment of surgeons." He asked to be reappointed with the understanding that he would consent to take the examination; he did so, passed, and was reappointed.[11]

It is difficult to determine how many medical officers resigned rather than submit to examination, since reasons for resignation were usually not included in official records. One example, however, was Surgeon E. B. Turnipseed, who had received awards and testimonials for his service on the Russian side during the Crimean War. "Fortified by these credentials in addition to his original diploma," reported a Charleston newspaper, "Dr. Turnipseed deemed it unnecessary and improper to submit to re-examination before an Army Medical Board. He conceived that the appointment of an Examining Board involved some discrimination, and was only designed to apply to cases of new appointments from civil life, and to young and unknown surgeons." Learning that he could not escape being examined, he resigned. The potential humiliation of failure certainly accounted for the resistance of some medical officers. A Richmond newspaper recognized that concern soon after the first boards were formed, anticipated that some surgeons and assistant surgeons would be judged unqualified, and attempted to soothe the bruised egos of those so found by ensuring them that "the jurisdiction of these boards has no reference whatever to the civil reputation of the gentlemen brought before them."[12]

Examinations and Prerequisites

Examinees were required to demonstrate their medical knowledge by writing responses to written questions and then responding orally to questions posed in person by members of the board. According to instructions from the SGO, those evaluating medical officers were to scrutinize the examinees' "moral and professional acquirements" and were expected to make a favorable report "in all cases which will admit of a reasonable belief that the officer will be able to meet the demands on his professional information." Examinations of medical officers were to be "practical, liberal, and so eminently fair as to give none the right to complain," while those of new applicants were to be "rigid in the professional requirements, as they have no right to complain of any standard which may be adopted." The SGO indicated, "it is intended that the examination of the Medical Officers of high reputation, Professors in Medical Schools, and others of Known merit will be a matter of form." Board decisions were to be communicated to the examinees. New applicants who passed received an appointment when their services were needed. Medical officers who failed and did not resign immediately were dropped from the army rolls.[13]

Assistant surgeons in the PACS could apply for promotion if they had practiced medicine for at least five years—in contrast with the five years of service at their current rank required of assistant surgeons in the regular Confederate army. Exceptions could be made for those applying for a vacancy in their regiment. At times assistant surgeons were urged by superior officers to apply for promotion and took the examination, although it is unclear whether those individuals always had five years of practice experience. Unsuccessful candidates had to wait at least six months before being examined a second time. In some cases men who had the rank of surgeon before being examined were recommended by a board for the rank of assistant surgeon and were subsequently demoted.[14]

Examinees were instructed to indicate, on their application, where and when they had graduated from medical school, but the extent to which graduation—or even attendance—was formally required is unclear. Confidential instructions from the SGO to the Knoxville board in October 1862 did not mention medical school, but similar instructions to the Chattanooga board in March 1863 bore a statement, looking much like an afterthought, below the surgeon general's signature: "All medical officers and applicants must be graduates of a respectable medical school. They will be interrogated on the subject." Thus, a graduation requirement may have been formalized halfway through the war after being applied inconsistently, or not at all, up to that point. Consistent with that possibility is the experience of Charles W. Trueheart, who had completed a term of medical school at the University of Virginia in early 1861, served as a Confederate infantryman and artillerist, performed the duties of an assistant surgeon in hospitals, and applied (probably in mid-1863) for a commission as assistant surgeon. That request, said Trueheart, was "refused by the Surg Genl on the newly taken ground that I was not an M.D." Not all Confederate surgeons and assistant surgeons had a medical degree, and it is uncertain how often medical boards reported favorably on an examinee who lacked one. Thomas Fanning Wood, for example, began his first term at MCV in October 1862 and received an invitation in January 1863—before the term ended in March—to be examined by the Richmond board for an appointment as assistant surgeon. Wood's status as a medical student was known by Surgeon General Moore, who directed the issuance of the invitation, and by Surgeon Arthur E. Peticolas, a member of the Richmond board and one of Wood's instructors at MCV. Wood passed and was ordered in February to report for duty with the Army of Northern Virginia.[15]

Peticolas, unless he recused himself, would also have been on the board that in January 1862 examined—and found satisfactory—Surgeons Charles Bell Gibson and James Brown McCaw, fellow faculty members at MCV and surgeons in charge of Richmond's General Hospital No. 1 and Chimborazo Hospital, respectively. The two men's credentials most likely marked them as examinees for whom the process was "a matter of form." Another physician with impressive qualifications was Surgeon J. J. Chisolm, who had been professor of surgery at the Medical College of the State of South Carolina and had observed the practice of military medicine during the Second Italian War of Independence in 1859. His January 1862 examination in Charleston was judged favorably by a board headed by Surgeon Robert Alexander Kinloch, a fellow Charlestonian.[16]

Medical schools of the time typically offered a single series of lectures given by five to seven professors over a term lasting about five months (generally October–March). At any particular school, the lectures changed little, if at all, from year to year. Granting of a medical diploma required attendance of two terms, which did not necessarily have to be in consecutive years or even at the same school. Admission often required no more than the ability to pay the lecture fees, although apprenticeship experience was a prerequisite at some schools. Graduation requirements, and their rigor, varied and could include passing examinations, completing a thesis, and paying a fee. What constituted, in the surgeon general's mind, a "respectable medical school" is undetermined. Moore probably meant, at least, that the school taught regular (allopathic) medicine rather than an unorthodox or sectarian system, such as homeopathy, botanical medicine, or Thomsonian medicine. W. T. Park, a botanical physician, asserted that the Medical Department was entirely controlled by allopaths and "ruled with a tyrannical power, not allowing any showing whatever to the Reform or Botanical Profession," whose ascendancy it feared. "The Surg. Gen'l will tell you that the existing board will examine any applicant and show no partiality," he continued. "I know them and the Surg. Gen'l too to be so prejudiced and so alarmed for the safety of their own craft that it would be impossible."[17]

Perceived Fairness and Effectiveness of Examinations

As would be expected, the operations of medical boards drew criticism. The panel at Charleston, South Carolina, was accused of favoring the interests of the medical college there, as evidenced by "the unusual number of medical students sporting the Confederate uniform about the hospitals of Charleston." (The Medical College of the State of South Carolina, in Charleston, closed after spring 1861.) Assistant Surgeon J. Hume Simons, after failing his examination there, asserted that board members, faced with more applicants than positions to fill, "claimed the right of selecting their favored applicants, to the rejection of those already appointed by the President, of whom I was one." Simons declined an offer by Surgeon General Moore to be reexamined by the Richmond board and resigned his position. Surgeon Edward Warren, a member of the board at Goldsboro, North Carolina, complained that the chairman applied the too-rigid standards of the US Army and was biased against North Carolinians. Warren declined to identify the chairman, but he was probably South Carolinian Nathaniel S. Crowell, surgeon in the PACS, assistant surgeon in the regular Confederate army, and former assistant surgeon in the US Army. The surgeon general evidently questioned whether the board at Little Rock, Arkansas, was too lax. On the contrary, said its president, Surgeon Philip O. Hooper, the board's standards were "thought by many of the old army surgeons too rigid, considering the available material." Hooper could not address the truth of a charge that his panel had passed applicants who had been rejected by the Mississippi board. Phoebe Yates Pember, a matron at Chimborazo Hospital, complained about a surgeon who had been a barkeeper and dispensary clerk before he came to Richmond, where the examining board approved him "by a process known only to themselves, which often rejected good practitioners, and gave appointments to apothecary boys." A writer to a Macon newspaper asserted that an applicant had only "to get a smattering of the healing art" from a textbook and that it did not matter "whether you have ever seen the inside of a Medical College, or attended hospitals or Cliniques." Josiah Nott, a one-time hopeful for the office of Confederate surgeon general and a board member at Mobile, described the application process as tedious and taking too long to assign successful applicants to positions. "The Board is useful in keeping out incompetent officers," he said, "but beyond this, is useless."[18]

Even individuals who had passed a board examination expressed reservations. Aristides Monteiro, who served as a medical officer under cavalryman John S. Mosby, described his examination as "not difficult but peculiar" and attacked the qualifications and beliefs of most members of the examining board. Ferdinand E. Daniel, not yet twenty-three years old and less than six months from having received a medical degree, was surprised to learn that his examination performance had earned him an appointment as a full surgeon and an immediate assignment as secretary to an examining board. Simon Baruch described passing a "rigid examination" when not yet twenty-two years old and being appointed assistant surgeon for five hundred soldiers "before ever having treated a sick person or ever having lanced a boil."[19]

The work of the examining boards had its defenders too. At the end of 1861, three months after establishment of the first panels, Secretary of War Benjamin reported that "happy effects have already resulted from the general examination by medical boards of the surgical staff of the Army." Many medical officers were "unequal to the duties of their station," some "were found incompetent from carelessness and neglect," and others displayed "gross ignorance of the very elements of the profession." Benjamin concluded that "the efficiency of the corps has been greatly increased by the purgation it has undergone." Moore, in a postwar address, characterized the system of examinations as "highly satisfactory." Stanford E. Chaillé, who had served on a board associated with the Army of Tennessee, acknowledged that the dismissal of medical officers sometimes "incurred the hostility of the officers and men in consequence." He attributed that reaction to "the gross incompetence of laymen . . . to judge of the incompetence of medical men." With regard to such dismissals, a Richmond newspaper opined, "it is better that some of the skillful should be lost than that all of the unskillful should be retained."[20]

Although an overall turnover rate for medical officers has never been determined, it was quite common for positions to be vacated because of their holders' inability to pass the board examination, chronic illness, physical disability, promotion, or another reason. Because departing medical officers had to be replaced, any particular position—say, assistant surgeon for a specific regiment—on average, was occupied by more than one individual during the course of the war. Thus, examining boards kept busy evaluating men already appointed as surgeon or assistant surgeon as well as new applicants for vacated positions.

Addressing Competence in Practice

Passage of an examination did not guarantee sound clinical judgment, so the surgeon general instructed medical directors of hospitals to form, at each hospital station, "a board of medical officers, to be consulted by the surgeon in charge in all important surgical cases, or when an operation is deemed necessary." When it was possible to wait, Moore directed that the panel approve all important surgical operations. Since so many medical officers had little or no surgical experience in their recent civilian practice, incorporating the opinions of more seasoned surgeons seemed prudent.[21]

Medical directors were allowed, when necessary, to employ civilian physicians as so-called contract surgeons. Although Medical Department regulations were silent on the specific qualifications necessary, Surgeon General Moore instructed in April 1863 that "the utmost care should be taken to appoint none but the deserving. Contracts are not to be made with young men. If they cannot pass an examination, they are not worthy of the position and their contracts should be cancelled." He ordered medical directors in December 1863 not to employ any physician whose examination before a medical board— either as a medical officer or an applicant to become a medical officer—had been unsatisfactory. The surgeon general was also indignant that some contract surgeons were dressing as medical officers. Moore instructed medical directors to disseminate the information that regulations did not allow such men to wear the uniform of officers appointed in the medical corps "in order that those who have adopted this unauthorized practice may abandon it."[22]

Examination of Hospital Stewards

Moore also applied an examination system to hospital stewards, noncommissioned officers whose responsibilities could include preparing medicines, assisting surgeons in the field or with surgical procedures, and supervising various functions in general hospitals. A steward could be appointed from the ranks of enlisted soldiers and, according to regulations, was not to be recommended for an appointment unless "*known* to be temperate, honest, and in every way reliable, as well as sufficiently intelligent, and skilled in pharmacy, for the proper discharge of the responsible duties likely to be devolved upon him." In August 1863 Moore instructed medical directors of hospitals to establish medical boards to "enquire into the competency and moral fitness of all Hospital Stewards within their jurisdiction, as well as the necessity for their employment in the department."[23]

Little is known about how effectively this order was carried out. Records exist for a board established by Surgeon Carrington in Virginia. He formed a panel of three surgeons to examine all hospitals stewards assigned to general hospitals in the state and instructed them to hold daily examining sessions in Richmond. Its members were to determine the stewards' physical capacity, moral fitness, intelligence, and skill required to perform their duties; also to be considered were testimonials from officers under whom the hospital stewards had served. Carrington instructed the board to classify examinees as those who were fully qualified; those who were not skilled in pharmacy but were able to perform important tasks and whose services were necessary, possibly as mess stewards or clerks; and those who were unqualified and not needed. One hospital steward concerned about the examination was George W. Sites, stationed at a general hospital in Lynchburg, Virginia, who thought himself unqualified in pharmacy beyond preparing "powders and potions." He also detested Surgeon Carrington, thought the feeling was mutual, and believed that Carrington would ensure his failure.[24]

Training for Future Medical Officers

Historians have placed the number of US allopathic medical schools in 1860 at forty-seven, with fifteen of those located in the states that would join the Confederacy. After the 1860–61 academic term, most of those fifteen closed, and only five had graduates for the terms ending in 1862–65: MCV, the New Orleans School of Medicine, the University of Louisiana, the University of Nashville, and the University of Virginia. The Union capture of New Orleans prompted the closure of the two Louisiana schools after the 1861–62 term, and the University of Virginia had only 5 medical graduates in 1862–65. Despite the Union occupation of Nashville, the medical school there remained open and had 75 graduates in 1862–65. MCV led the way with 191 medical graduates in 1862–65. Not only did MCV remain open, but its hospital also was used to care for Confederate soldiers, while its faculty members became Confederate surgeons or otherwise assisted in Richmond hospitals. Surgeon General Moore saw the value of MCV as a training facility for future medical officers and arranged for selected individuals—usually hospital stewards or soldiers with such duties—to be posted to general hospitals in Richmond and to attend lectures at MCV. "On graduation," he remembered, "letters of invitation were issued them for examination for appointment [as medical officers] in the corps."[25]

As was illustrated by MCV student Thomas Fanning Wood, graduation was not always a prerequisite for appearance before a board and appointment as a medical officer. Perhaps Moore's familiarity with the school's solid reputation, his experience with MCV professor McCaw in establishing Chimborazo Hospital, and the presence of MCV professor Peticolas on Richmond's examining board allowed a loosening of the graduation requirement for certain of its students. Others who graduated under Moore's plan had already completed one term of medical school before entering the army. For example, James T. Meek attended the 1860–61 lectures of the Medical College of the State of South Carolina, graduated from MCV after attending its 1862–63 session, received a favorable evaluation from the examination board in Charleston, and was appointed as assistant surgeon. The aforementioned Trueheart, after completing a session of medical lectures elsewhere, graduated from MCV after the 1863–64 term, received a favorable report from the Richmond board, and was appointed as assistant surgeon.[26]

The number of MCV graduates appointed as medical officers in the Confederate army was relatively small—fifty-nine for the graduating classes of 1861–64 combined. The precise contribution of the school in preparing enlisted personnel to be army surgeons is difficult to determine, in part because it is uncertain exactly when Surgeon General Moore began sending those men there and how many MCV-trained medical officers were in the army before attending its medical lectures. And as mentioned above, some men who attended MCV became medical officers without having received a medical diploma. Nevertheless, the initiative was innovative and resourceful, rewarded high-performing enlisted medical personnel, and added medical officers to the Confederate army in numbers that would at least help replace surgeons who resigned, failed examinations before medical boards, or otherwise left the army. It also illustrated Moore's awareness that new medical graduates were scarce and his working assumption that the war would continue.[27]

Securing competent medical personnel in adequate numbers challenged the Medical Department throughout the war. But there also existed the need to educate new army surgeons about military medicine and to relay even to experienced medical officers the lessons being learned on the field and in hospitals. That need was partially met by providing written information and by collecting and analyzing reports sent to the SGO.

12. Adding to Medical Knowledge

The SGO spent considerable effort disseminating information to medical officers in the field and hospitals. Collecting data from those same officers was a priority, not only because it had been standard practice in the US Army—and the Confederate SGO was controlled by traditionalists recently in that army—but also because the value of the data to current and future practitioners (and to historians) was well understood.

Books as Educational Tools

Most new Confederate medical officers were inexperienced in establishing healthful camp conditions, treating battlefield wounds, or managing the illnesses to which large groups of men were prone. Furthermore, as former Confederate surgeon Henry F. Campbell observed, "the difficulties of communication attending the blockade rendered it impossible to supply the army with convenient and suitable medical works." In November 1861 Medical Director and Purveyor Alexander N. Talley told a medical officer, "Medical books cannot be had & their distribution [is] disallowed on the grounds of their cost & scarcity." That state of affairs prompted Southern publishers to reprint Northern textbooks. *A Manual of Military Surgery; or, Hints on the Emergencies of Field, Camp and Hospital Practice*, by renowned Philadelphia surgeon Samuel D. Gross, was first published in late May 1861 by Philadelphia's Lippincott and Company. The short work, meant to be a practical and portable reference, was reproduced, except for its appendix, in the July and August 1861 issues of the *Southern Medical and Surgical Journal*, based in Augusta, Georgia. It was also reproduced as a book in 1861 by the *Augusta Chronicle & Sentinel* and in 1862 by J. W. Randolph in Richmond. There is no evidence that those copies were undertaken at the request of the Confederate government, although they would have been useful for appointed or potential medical officers.[1]

A book that got similar treatment was *Notes on the Surgery of the War in Crimea*, by George H. B. Macleod, first published in 1858 in London.

A smaller version—185 pages, compared with the original 439 pages—was edited by Talley, who was forced to abridge the work to accommodate "the narrowed resources of the times." His edition was published in mid-1862 in Richmond by J. W. Randolph and did not indicate any involvement of the surgeon general.[2]

Surgeon J. J. Chisolm contributed *A Manual of Military Surgery, for the Use of Surgeons in the Confederate States Army*, with editions published in 1861, 1862, and 1864. In the third edition, released in mid-1864, Chisolm acknowledged the assistance provided by the SGO in providing statistics but never implied that the work had been prepared at the request or order of Surgeon General Moore. The print run of that edition was fewer than two thousand copies, and by December 1864 publisher Evans and Cogswell was hoping that the government would buy as many as nine hundred copies still on hand. Edward Warren's *Epitome of Practical Surgery, for Field and Hospital* was written and published in 1863 after the author resigned his commission as a Confederate surgeon to become surgeon general of North Carolina. Both Chisolm and Warren acknowledged borrowing content from other works. The books by Macleod, Chisolm, and Warren were said to have been in common use by Confederate surgeons.[3]

Moore said in 1875 that he had assigned medical officers to write treatises on military surgery and on injuries to the nerves. The former was likely what a medical officer, probably from the SGO, described when he told a Richmond newspaper in November 1863 that "an accomplished physiologist and pathologist has been relieved of all other duties, and every facility is being afforded him for preparing a compend of surgery." It appears that neither treatise mentioned in Moore's postwar remarks was published during the war.[4]

The surgeon general also directed the preparation of a field book on operative surgery, which materialized as *A Manual of Military Surgery, Prepared for the Use of the Confederate States Army*, published in late 1863 in Richmond. The book was created by a group of medical officers who, "unambitious of authorship," declined to identify themselves. They called the book "a brief collection of papers" based on material published elsewhere and supplemented with remarks reflecting their own experience. According to the one postwar source, the compilers were understood to have been Surgeons Talley, Campbell, St. George Peachy, Arthur E. Peticolas, and James Dunn, a supposition consistent with a wartime statement that the authors were members of Richmond's medical examining board. (The five men were on the board but not all at the same time.) The involvement of Campbell seems certain from contemporary accounts, and a biographical sketch of Talley mentions his participation, but there is little or no solid documentation that Peachy, Peticolas, and Dunn were also among the compilers. The book was evidently widely distributed among Confederate medical officers, with more than four hundred copies distributed among those of the Army of Tennessee.[5]

Probably the best-known publication produced at the surgeon general's direction was Surgeon Francis Peyre Porcher's *Resources of the Southern Fields and Forests*. As part of Moore's encouragement of medical officers to use preparations of indigenous plants as medicines, the SGO distributed a twenty-two-page pamphlet on April 2, 1862, (its official issue date was March 21) that instructed surgeons how such plants were to be collected and prepared. The pamphlet, whose authorship is unknown, listed sixty-seven useful species with instructions for dosage for each and the disorders for which they were useful. But its conciseness robbed it of detail, and its descriptions of the plants were probably too sparse to ensure that the correct flora would be collected. On May 27, 1863, Moore ordered Porcher, who had a special interest in Southern botany, "to proceed to South Carolina to superintend the forming of a botanical garden" and to "supervise and enlarge the pamphlet." Why a garden was desired is unclear, but he may have wanted it to contain reference samples of plants positively identified by Porcher as useful for medicinal purposes. In June 1862 Moore approved Porcher's plans for the garden and told him, "After your *pamphlet* [emphasis added] shall have been finished, and the garden in operation, you can be assigned to hospital duty."[6]

By January 1863 Charleston publisher Evans and Cogswell had started converting Porcher's manuscript into print, and in March the finished product, *Resources of the Southern Fields and Forests*, was complete and ready for sale and shipping. Instead of a pamphlet, Porcher's final product was a 601-page book that described how preparations of indigenous plants could be used not only medicinally but also in the production of cloth, cordage, dyes, fertilizer, paper, and other items useful in the "domestic economy." To Surgeon William A. Carrington, medical director of Virginia general hospitals, the book sounded promising, so he asked Moore to provide a copy for each of the state's thirty-three hospitals outside of Richmond. Being produced with the surgeon general's sanction, he said, would ensure the book being read, and its suggestions were sure to save the government some money.[7]

The book was praised by newspapers, but its medicinal content might just as easily have been compiled and reprinted from other available sources. Porcher had arranged plants taxonomically and did not clearly indicate the preparations preferred for particular symptoms or disorders. Joseph St. Julien Guerard, a Charleston physician, appreciated the effort but considered the book "crude, imperfect and unsatisfactory." According to Guerard, who offered his comments in October 1864, "the medical staff of the Army, for whom it was primarily intended, make little use of it. They complain (and justly too) that as no botanical or physical description is given of the different plants treated of, and no plates exhibited, they remain just as much in the dark as they were before, and the Doctor's labor, therefore, thrown away, as far as they are concerned." *Resources* was also expensive. Evans and Cogswell charged the government $2.37 per unbound copy and $2.97 per bound copy. Richmond's West and Johnston, which also released *Resources*—its version was actually printed in Charleston by Evans and Cogswell—established a retail price of $10.00. That contrasted with the much lower prices charged in 1863 for the aforementioned books by Gross ($1.00), Macleod ($1.75), Chisolm ($4.00), and Warren ($5.00) and in 1864 for the Moore-ordered, anonymously written *Manual* ($6.00). On March 1, 1863, to coincide with the availability of *Resources*, the SGO issued the *Standard Supply Table of the Indigenous Remedies*, which enumerated the amounts of plant-based remedies to be kept by units in the field and in general hospitals. Of the sixty-five species in the new table, fifty-eight had already appeared in the March 1862 pamphlet.[8]

Moore said in 1875 that the pamphlet on indigenous plants "did not meet the requirements of the army or the necessities of the people of the Confederacy. It seemed incumbent to furnish the latter with all the information and practical instruction possible." Furthermore, he noted, Porcher's book "was of so much importance, containing a great deal of valuable and useful information, that a large edition was published and the volumes distributed free to those who desired them." The pamphlet, however, had clearly been prepared for medical officers rather than the public, and educating the latter by providing Porcher's book gratis—if such giveaways actually occurred—seems inconsistent with Moore's scope of responsibility and his need to be frugal with his department's financial and intellectual resources. If *Resources* did not meet the surgeon general's expectations, he was probably reluctant to publicly criticize Porcher, a respected physician and fellow South Carolinian. And if the book was actually more useful to the public than to medical officers, then framing it as having been prepared largely for public consumption conveniently accounted for why *Resources* turned out as it did. It is unclear why it was advertised for sale if it was indeed given away to anyone who desired a copy. At Moore's urging, newspapers printed excerpts—no doubt selected by the SGO—from *Resources* that described natural products that might be medicinally useful to the army or the community.[9]

Gathering Knowledge

Moore knew that medical officers in the field and in general hospitals were amassing valuable clinical experience. As a way of gathering and synthesizing that practical knowledge, and perhaps drawing conclusions from it, he encouraged the formation of the Association of Army and Navy Surgeons (AANS). The group, whose first official session was on August 22, 1863, met at MCV and was open to all medical officers in the Confederate army and navy who signed the AANS constitution and contributed ten dollars as well as to various honorary members, such as MCV faculty who were not in the military. Sessions were intended to occur every two weeks, with written submissions on and open discussion of predetermined topics. Moore was elected president of AANS and served through the organization's existence. The group's final session was on March 18, 1865.[10]

Discussion questions proposed by Moore were distributed to medical officers via SGO circulars in five series—the first four issued during the latter half of 1863 and the fifth on February 27, 1864. Those topics dealt with surgical concerns, such as the nature and healing of gunshot wounds, the use of chloroform, shock, hemorrhage, and amputation, but discussion at the biweekly meetings could entail other subjects, such as smallpox vaccination and the ideal characteristics of military hospitals. Thomas Fanning Wood recalled attending one of the meetings: "I was but a looker on, attracted by a sight of the men whose names I had often heard." In addition to the surgeon general, the attendees mentioned by Wood included Surgeons Chisolm, William Middleton Michel, and Edwin S. Gaillard. The meetings resembled a weekly "quiz class" organized at Richmond's Winder Hospital by its director, Surgeon Alexander G. Lane. There, a seven-member faculty of Lane and division surgeons conducted lessons for the facility's medical officers on assigned topics, with the result that "all were refreshed in both theory and daily practice, drawn together both socially and intellectually." According to Lane, attendees "passed with flying colors before the Army Examining Board, and thirty-three assistant surgeons in Winder Hospital were promoted to full surgeons."[11]

Moore understood how reports from the field and from hospitals could inform the SGO of trends in soldiers' health and lessons learned in the management of disease and wounds. Thus, not only did he assign Surgeon Joseph

Jones to gather data about various maladies of soldiers and prisoners but also insisted that medical officers follow regulations and his own directives about recording and submitting detailed information. Those officers, lacking a military background and disdaining red tape, were often delinquent in such tasks. In a June 1862 circular, Moore chastised surgeons for failing to keep adequate records on gunshot wounds and their treatment and explained the need for their compliance: "This is demanded not only in justice to the corps of which they are members, and from which much interesting and useful statistical information will be expected at the close of the war, but also for the benefit of the science of surgery at large, which should not be robbed of the advantages supposed to accrue from so extended a field of observation as that which now presents itself."[12] In April 1863 the surgeon general issued another circular, this time bemoaning "the frequency with which Reports of the Sick and Wounded reach this office incomplete and defective, and wholly unsuited to establish accurate and reliable statistics concerning the prevalence of disease throughout the army."[13]

The prevention of smallpox was of particular concern to the surgeon general, and he searched for ways to procure safe vaccine matter and to understand the worrisome phenomenon known as spurious vaccination, in which inoculated patients developed abnormal lesions. Vaccine matter was ideally obtained from cows with cowpox lesions but could also be taken from the lesion of humans already vaccinated. Spurious vaccination was thought to be related to material that was tainted or improperly collected, especially when taken from humans. Thus, Moore directed hospital surgeons "to report all cases of patients who are afflicted with a particularly annoying and disgusting disease, produced, it is supposed, by the use of impure or spurious vaccine virus." When Surgeon John D. Jackson of the Army of Tennessee submitted a report titled "Spurious Vaccination or Phagadaemic Ulceration Following Vaccination," Moore noted that the disorder seemed identical to one prevalent in the Army of Northern Virginia and ordered the Army of Tennessee's medical director to identify "intelligent observers" among his surgeons to submit "extended and critical reports" concerning spurious vaccination among their patients.[14]

In early 1862, the surgeon general, on learning of a cowpox-like disease called "grease," which was afflicting cavalry horses and was communicable to humans, wondered whether the equine disease was related to cowpox. He thus directed Surgeon Thomas H. Williams of the Army of the Potomac to conduct an experiment. Vaccine matter collected from cavalry troopers afflicted by handling diseased horses would be administered to cows to see if disease developed; if so, those cows could be a source of vaccine matter to be given to soldiers. Williams had the experiment conducted, but its results are unknown. The next year, surgeons in the Army of Northern Virginia discussed inoculating cows with vaccine matter—presumably from humans—so that fresh and reliable vaccine matter could be harvested from the resulting bovine lesions. Moore's collection of information considered useful "as well in a practical as a scientific point of view" contributed to practices and procedures that he imposed on medical officers. An October 1863 circular from the SGO, for example, sought to avoid "the pernicious results which have followed the careless employment of impure virus in vaccinating the army" by providing detailed instructions on collecting and administering vaccine material. Moore also ordered surgeons to "vaccinate gratis the healthy children in the vicinity" of their posting so that the resultant lesions would constitute "a fresh supply of pure vaccine virus." The latter was a rare example of military surgeons providing medical care to civilians, albeit with a motive of assisting the army.[15]

The *Confederate States Medical and Surgical Journal*

In the fall of 1863, Richmond's *Southern Illustrated News* noted the absence of published medical information about and from the army, accused the SGO of indifference in collecting such data, and urged its presentation in a new medical journal. In response, an anonymous correspondent—who called himself "Surgeon" and was almost certainly from the SGO—acknowledged the "necessity for the establishment of such a periodical, conducted under the authority of the Government, and used exclusively for the publication of results elicited by elaborate and carefully prepared statistics." Within the past eighteen months, added the correspondent, "a separate department has been organized and placed in charge of competent medical officers, whose sole duty consists in arranging, tabulating and indexing the vast amount of information" in reports submitted to the SGO by field and hospital surgeons. Noted military surgeons of the past had furnished "the profession generally with the results of their experience—and such is the intention of Southern surgeons." Those renowned physicians "collected, compared and revised their field and hospital notes, and published them, *at the close of the war*," and such, asserted the correspondent, "is the intention of Southern surgeons." The response concluded grandly: "Revolutions in surgical science—the result of the investigations of Southern surgeons—are taking place, that will overthrow the hitherto accepted dogmas of European authors; and theories are being established by an overwhelming array of carefully digested facts, that will, when published, redeem them from the charge of somnolence and slothfulness."[16]

While AANS was being organized and the *Southern Illustrated News* was printing the exchange above, plans formed in Richmond to publish a medical journal. The war crisis and the imposition of a blockade had largely deprived Southern physicians of current medical literature. "In the Southern States," observed a wartime Northern medical publication, "once so prolific in medical periodicals that each considerable town had one or more representatives, the whole serial medical literature has long since disappeared." Thus, Richmond's Ayres and Wade, "with the hearty approval of the Surgeon-General," commenced publishing the *Confederate States Medical and Surgical Journal (CSMSJ)* in January 1864. The monthly journal was to assist the medical officers of the Confederate military "to lay before the world the results of its labor," act in concert with AANS, and reprint pertinent European medical literature. The editors stated that "with free access to the archives and reports of the Medical Department, and with the approval and under the supervision of the Surgeon-General, the vast statistics and tabulated records of the war can be carefully collated and made to subserve their legitimate uses." According to Ayres and Wade, *CSMSJ* operated under the direction of Surgeon James B. McCaw, an experienced medical-journal editor who had worked with the surgeon general to establish Chimborazo Hospital. Surgeon Michel also appears to have had a role in editing the periodical. The extent to which Moore influenced the journal's content in unknown.[17]

CSMSJ, which published its last issue in February 1865, featured case reports and other contributions from medical officers, AANS proceedings, occasional summaries of medical statistics provided by the SGO, reprints of Northern and European publications, and official listings of selected army medical personnel and facilities. By May 1864 the journal's editor reported that it had "already attained a larger circulation than was ever reached before by any Southern medical periodical." The annual subscription fee was ten dollars (in advance) but rose to twenty dollars in September 1864 because of growing labor and paper costs. That increase was accompanied by an expansion in issue size from sixteen pages through August 1864 to twenty-four pages thereafter. Some of the additional space was devoted to expanded coverage of foreign literature, which was made possible by the editor "having successfully opened a regular communication with the European journals." The increase in issue length fell short of the doubling (to thirty-two pages) that the editor hoped to achieve to accommodate "the wealth of material, both original and selective," on hand and awaiting publication.[18]

Analyzing Data in the SGO

The SGO department that "Surgeon" had described as "arranging, tabulating and indexing" clinical information was composed of Surgeons Francis Sorrel and Herman Baer. Edward Warren, in his *Epitome of Practical Surgery*, cited Sorrel's careful collection of statistics under the "intelligent scrutiny and able direction" of Surgeon General Moore. Chisolm, in the 1864 edition of his *Manual of Military Surgery*, gave special credit to Baer: "I am under heavy obligation to my friend, Surgeon H. Baer, P.A.C.S., who was kindly permitted by Surgeon F. Sorrel, C.S.A., the accomplished and efficient Inspector-General of Hospitals, to collate for me condensed tabulated reports of all the hospital and field surgeons of the Confederate army. Only those who have undertaken to tabulate statistics can appreciate the labor of Surgeon Baer." Sorrel, lamenting the loss of records in Richmond's evacuation fire, said that they "would have proved a noble testimony to the high professional skill and success of our surgeons." In an 1875 address, Moore uttered "love's labor lost" to describe his sorrow about the fate of the records he labored so hard to collect. "It is much to be regretted that the public documents belonging to our department have been lost or destroyed," he said. "I apprehend much difficulty will be experienced by those . . . [tasked with making] reports on various subjects connected with the medical history of the war, for without the necessary data perfect reports cannot be made or expected."[19]

Moore's Contribution

In striving to make the knowledge of experienced practitioners widely available, Surgeon General Moore ordered the preparation of various publications, which were supplemented by other efforts (such as the reprints of Gross and the texts by Chisolm and Warren) apparently undertaken independently of his desires. Whether the SGO could have pursued a more vigorous publishing agenda, especially in the latter half of the war, when inflation was particularly rampant, is unclear. Rising costs forced *CSMSJ* to double its subscription price in the fall of 1864 after just seven months of publication. Evans and Cogswell, publisher of Chisolm's and Porcher's books, noted in late 1864 that the Confederate currency system and the escalating cost of paper—especially imported paper, on which most of their books were printed—resulted in their losing money with every copy sold at prices they had set only five months earlier. Even if Moore had additional information he wanted published, it might have been impossible to do so at an affordable price.[20]

The surgeon general also encouraged discussion of important medical and surgical topics through the AANS and likely hoped that any vital conclusions might be communicated to field and hospital surgeons in time to ameliorate the suffering of sick or wounded soldiers. Medical histories of the war suffer from a want of extensive Confederate statistics, but this is attributable to the loss of records as the war ended, not to a failure on Moore's part to accumulate them. All in all, the actions taken by the SGO to educate its officers and collect data from them were vigorous and commendable.

13. ✳ Examining for Disability

onfederate medical officers became involved in boards other than those examining medical officers and applicants. The army's huge need for manpower and the waning of volunteering after the winter of 1861–62 prompted the initiation of conscription and necessitated measures to keep able-bodied men who were already in the army from leaving under the guise of disability. At the same time, truly infirm men—who would be a burden to the army while contributing little to its fighting strength—had to be excluded. As the war progressed, such measures were altered to expand the pool of conscripts (by widening the age range of eligible men) and make evasion of active military service more difficult. Those changes, both frequent and complex, are described here to the extent that they involved the Medical Department. Its major contributions were the assignment of medical officers to conduct the required examinations, the advice evidently provided by the surgeon general regarding the health-related conditions that justified exemptions for disability, and the granting of medical furloughs, leaves of absence, and discharges.

Examining Conscripts and Granting Details

Troops for the Confederate army were initially supplied by the individual Southern states though their own recruiting systems. On April 16, 1862, President Davis approved the First Conscription Act, which made all men between the ages of eighteen and thirty-five years and residing in the Confederate States subject to military service. The president was empowered, with the consent of the individual states, to employ state officials in enrollment activities or, lacking that permission, to employ Confederate personnel to do the same in accordance with rules and regulations that he would prescribe. How Confederate medical officers might be involved was not immediately clear, but on April 28 the AIGO provided some guidance. It indicted that an army officer would be assigned to each state "to take charge of the enrollment, mustering in, subsistence, transportation and disposition of the Recruits raised under the above act." If the government was not allowed by a state to employ state officers in enrollment, Confederate army officers would be assigned those duties. Substitutes—individuals otherwise exempt from duty but willing to serve in place of nonexempt men—would be accepted only after being pronounced sound by a surgeon or assistant surgeon.[1]

Two days later the AIGO directed that "the Regulations already in force for ascertaining physical ability or disability for military service, are continued." Those regulations instructed:

> In passing a recruit, the medical officer is to examine him stripped; to see that he has free use of his limbs; that his chest is ample; that his hearing, vision, and speech are perfect; that he has no tumors, or ulcerations or extensively cicatrized legs; no rupture, or chronic cutaneous affection; that he has not received any contusion, or wound of the head, which may impair his faculties; that he is not a drunkard; is not subject to convulsions, and has no infectious disorder, nor any other that may unfit him for military service.[2]

By July 1862, Confederate medical officers were examining recruits. In Georgia such duty was being performed at Augusta, Savannah, Macon, and Camp Randolph (near Calhoun). In a circular that month, Surgeon General Moore supplemented the instructions provided in the regulations. Medical officers examining recruits, he said, should not be rejecting men with "trivial defects" but should pass anyone "capable of bearing arms." Furthermore, a recruit should not be rejected solely by presenting "a certificate of disability from any medical man." Instead, "such certificates should come from a medical officer designated or detailed" for the examination of recruits. In this last specification, Moore was trying to avoid a situation described earlier in 1862 by Virginia governor John Letcher after the commonwealth had enacted an exemption law. Letcher noted the "startling" number of exemptions, which he attributed to the fact that "each man who desires to procure exemption is permitted to seek the physicians he deems most facile to grant certificates, and by paying them fees for examination a mere nominal and verbal examination is made."[3]

Contrary to instructions, certificates provided by civilian physicians were being accepted by Confederate enrolling officers in Georgia, a situation that forced Major John Dunwody, commandant of Camp Randolph, to mandate that the improperly exempted men reappear to be examined by an approved surgeon. Instead of applying the relatively liberal exceptions suggested in army regulations, Surgeon General Moore instructed examining surgeons to assume that "all men are supposed to be capable of performing military duty who are able to perform the common avocations of life, and whose disability is not so great as to make them useless as farmers or daily laborers." According to Dunwody, the old-army regulations were intended for a time of peace, when "only perfect men were then received," but the current situation was different. "We desire fighting material," he said, "and have to take into service even those who may have to be discharged after a few months of service on account of weakness; still, for the time they are in the service, they will make good soldiers."[4]

An editorialist for Augusta's *Daily Constitutionalist* called Dunwody's pronouncements despotic and demanded to know "who constituted the Surgeon General, or Major Dunwoody [*sic*], and the enrolling officers generally, legislators, to alter the old system of examinations and exemptions, and to establish new rules and new tests?" The authority, in fact, came directly from the War Department, as expressed in AIGO general orders on August 14, 1862. The directives indicated that at points where conscripts were gathered for enrollment and instruction, "an experienced Army Surgeon, from a different section of the country," would be detailed to examine conscripts. "All Conscripts capable of bearing arms will be received." Among allowable causes for exemption were "blindness, excessive deafness and permanent lameness, or great deformity" and "confirmed consumption, large incurable ulcers, and chronic contagious diseases of the skin." Disorders not considered grounds for dismissal included "single reducible hernia" and the "loss of an eye or of several fingers." Certificates of disability from private physicians were not to be considered unless accompanied by an affidavit that the subject was confined to bed or that his life would be endangered by travel to the place of enrollment. The names of conscripts found "not equal to all military duty" but able to perform valuable service in the various staff departments would be forwarded—with mention of previous occupation and recommendations for special duty—to the AIGO for appropriate assignment.[5]

The role of Confederate surgeons in examining conscripts was clarified further in an act approved on October 11, 1862, and in AIGO general orders specifying how the act was to be implemented. Places of rendezvous for enrollment of recruits would be manned by surgeons employed by the Confederate government and assigned by the president. Their decisions as to the fitness of conscripts to serve—under regulations established by the secretary of war—were final. Each congressional district would have a board of examiners consisting of three physicians, one of whom would be an army medical officer. The other two, civilians, would be recommended by the commandant of conscripts and come from districts different from that in which they examined conscripts. Any one or more of those physicians could act at any place of rendezvous in their assigned district. If the certificate of a respectable area physician stated that an enrollee could not appear because of infirmity, that man had to appear within a reasonable time and produce a certificate of continued disability or be considered absent without leave.[6]

Surgeon General Moore asked the AIGO in late November 1862 for a list of congressional districts, the identity of enrolling officers, and the location of points of rendezvous. How many assignments he had to make was not obvious. The Confederate Congress encompassed 106 districts from the eleven seceded states and the border states of Kentucky and Missouri; there were also nonvoting tribal and territorial delegates. Enrollment would not occur in all districts, and how the AIGO answered Moore is unknown, but the surgeon general quickly assigned medical officers to fill the specified roles. Between December 16, 1862, and January 6, 1863, for example, he designated surgeons for assignment to congressional districts in Alabama, Arkansas, Georgia, Mississippi, North Carolina, South Carolina, and Virginia.[7]

Moore probably had little to do with judging whether too many men were evading active field service, but he likely influenced orders issued by the AIGO in February 1863 that guided boards examining conscripts. Such panels, said the orders, "must exercise a sound and firm discretion, and not yield their judgment in favor of every complaint of trivial disability, by attaching too much attention to which, they indirectly favor evasions of the required military service." In general, men able to perform "all of the active duties of the various occupations of civilian life" should be able to become soldiers. The orders continued by listing conditions not warranting exemption, including general debility, slight deformity, deafness (unless serious enough "as to incapacitate a man for the duties of a sentinel"), impediment of speech, organic heart disease, functional disturbance of the heart's action (a "very common" condition "generally . . . relieved by change to the life of the camp"), rheumatism ("liable to be used as a means of evasion"), epilepsy ("frequently simulated"), varicocele, myopia ("many myopic subjects distinguish distant objects with accuracy sufficient for all practical purposes"), hemorrhoids, corneal opacity or loss of one eye, loss of one or two fingers, and single reducible hernia. It is unlikely than any of the top officers in the War Department other than the surgeon general could have created so specific a list. In February 1864 the

AIGO ordered that conscription boards, when possible, be composed of two medical officers and one civilian surgeon rather than the previously specified one medical officer and two civilian surgeons.[8]

The system of conscript examination and allowance of details was known to be faulty. In November 1864 Adjutant and Inspector General Cooper described the conscript medical boards as "subject to the suspicion of local and personal influence" and "charged with favoritism and other influences."[9] Harvey W. Walter, an AIGO inspector, regarded conscription in Georgia, Alabama, and Mississippi as "almost worthless." Walter observed in December that military posts were full of skulkers, men who generally appeared healthy but were nevertheless classified as disabled and thus detailed to work in the various military departments at the request of those departments:

> I approach a detail to every appearance sound, and he thrusts into my face a certificate of disability. . . . He looks strong enough to brain an ox with his knuckle and eat him afterward. . . . It is erroneous policy to force the question of fitness of details at a post upon the surgeons there. They are dependent upon the quartermaster there for home, office, fire, pay, clothing, and transportation, and receive from the commissary the food that feeds them. They would be less than human could they listen without prejudice to the petition of these officers for details, backed by assurances that they know the subject to be suffering from nearly "every ill that flesh is heir to." I could correct the evil could I see through the eyes of an intelligent physician not subject to these influences.[10]

In response to real and perceived abuses of the detail system, the AIGO revoked all details on October 8, with the exception of men "actually employed as artisans, mechanics or person of scientific skill (and those detailed and now engaged in the manufacture, collection and forwarding of indispensable supplies for the army and navy)." Heads of bureaus were to identify their detailed men who were experts, absolutely indispensable, and between eighteen and forty-five years old; men in that age range not absolutely indispensable would be assigned to the army, while those claiming disability would be examined by conscript boards. Later that month bureau chiefs were ordered to identify workers who were so indispensable as to be "exempt under all calls for military service except in the extreme emergency of an attack" upon Richmond. Although the surgeon general tried to protect his staff, the orders deprived him of some clerks and compromised the efficiency of his office.[11]

On March 7, 1865, President Davis approved an act—apparently prompted by a proposal from General Cooper—that transferred the control of conscription operations to generals of reserves in the various states. Conscripts would report to commands in the field and be examined by army medical boards of those units. Conscripts unable to join their assigned command because of disability would be furloughed until they could be examined by a board of three surgeons, two of whom would be Confederate medical officers; one such board was to be formed for each congressional district. Davis, in approving the act, urged its modification because it required—for examination of the small number of conscripts too disabled to join their command—the assignment of additional army surgeons. "After the first visit to the different counties," said Davis, "these officers would have so little to do as to be practically supernumeraries supported by the Government at great cost, and with the loss of their services in the field." The act effectively dissolved the previous conscription boards and, in doing so, allowed their medical officers—one or two per congressional district—to be reassigned to field or hospital duty. Davis thought that some 150 medical officers (two for each of about seventy-five districts with active recruiting) would be required by the act, probably constituting a net loss for the Medical Department in field and hospital surgeons. Congress repealed that provision of the act on March 17.[12]

Also on March 17 the AIGO ordered that soldiers detailed because of disability were to be examined monthly and conscripts assigned to light duty reexamined every three months; those found able would be sent to the field. The examinations were to be done by hospital medical boards—those formed to determine the need for furlough or discharge (as described later in this chapter)—or by conscript boards. Because the act of March 7 had abolished the conscript boards, perhaps those created by that law for examining furloughed conscripts were meant.[13]

Furloughs, Leaves of Absence, and Discharges

As procedures for the examination of recruits changed over time, so did those for granting medical furloughs, leaves, and discharges. (In army terminology "furloughs" pertained to enlisted men and "leaves of absence" to officers.) Early Confederate regulations for furloughs required a certificate from the senior surgeon of the hospital, regiment, or post. Obtaining the necessary approval required that the document be sent along a circuitous route. A modification of the process in November 1861 specified that the certificate be signed by the surgeon having charge of the invalid but still entailed delays that could essentially deny a timely furlough to a man who truly needed one. A committee of the House of Representatives noted the inefficiency of the existing system. For officers, medical leaves of absence required a certificate from the senior medical officer present; changes in legislation and regulations affecting furloughs typically did not address leaves of absence.[14]

On July 2, 1862, a special procedure was established for the Department of Henrico, which included Richmond. A board of three medical officers appointed by the surgeon general now would evaluate and report on all applications for medical furloughs, leaves of absence, and discharges. Certificates of disability were to be completed by medical officers attending the invalids or by "physicians of reputation" in the city; the latter, all civilians, might be caring for patients in private quarters. The board could approve an application if the disability was "decidedly and manifestly apparent" but would otherwise examine the patient. Board recommendations were to be approved, but the initial procedure did not say by whom. When a change of climate was necessary for the restoration of health, a passport to leave Richmond and transportation could be secured through the secretary of war. In early August 1862 Secretary Randolph ordered that each board member act separately in making examinations—in Moore's words, "destroying its character as a joint Board"—and that certificates of disability, when created by the examining members, were to be approved by Brigadier General John Winder, commander of the Department of Henrico.[15]

Members of Congress became aware of the Richmond panel but initially knew little about it, asking President Davis to explain. According to Senator James L. Orr of South Carolina, full surgeons in hospitals—who should best know the condition of their patients—resented having their certificates of disability second-guessed by assistant surgeons on the board. Representative Augustus R. Wright of Georgia claimed that the government refused to grant furloughs on the common belief that many soldiers, once away from the army, would not return. He considered such thinking libelous and claimed that furloughed men would return when they were able.[16]

Davis responded in late August 1862 by providing Congress with Surgeon General Moore's explanation. The board, said Moore, was the result of General Lee asking that the authority to grant furloughs be removed from surgeons in charge of hospitals and given instead to a single medical officer in Richmond, presumably the surgeon general. Because he could not run his department while attending to "such multitudes of applications as were then, and are yet, being made," Moore instead appointed a board, "which seems unfortunately to have given such offence to both branches of Congress." Lee's request stemmed from the fact that large numbers of certificates of disability were being forged. Moore's report suggested that the provost marshal and quartermaster, who issued passports and transportation tickets, were unfamiliar with the signatures of hospital surgeons and thus gave such documents to soldiers bearing certificates with forged signatures. He concluded by reporting that he had just formed similar boards at Chimborazo and Winder Hospitals, which were each large enough to justify having its own panel. Senator Orr was unimpressed, found Moore's explanation difficult to understand, and suggested that the surgeon general was deflecting blame from his own medical officers. Representative Hardy Strickland of Georgia proposed that the House's Special Committee on Hospitals look into abolishing the board.[17]

The system implemented, at Moore's direction, at Winder Hospital involved a panel of three division surgeons who examined applicants for furlough or discharge. The hospital's chief surgeon, Alexander G. Lane, approved the board's recommendations. Supplied with presigned passports and furloughs by the commander of the Department of Henrico, he could issue the documents directly and order transportation if needed. Lane reported that the arrangement worked admirably and allowed the invalid to begin his travels within a day of the furlough's approval. His comments, addressed to a congressional committee investigating the Medical Department (described below), may have provided a model for how the furlough system would develop.[18]

Continued congressional discussion in September 1862 about the original Richmond board—which had no jurisdiction over Winder or Chimborazo Hospitals—featured Representative William W. Clark of Georgia deriding the board members "as young and inexperienced—as a Board of boys." (The panel was indeed young, composed of Surgeon James H. Berrien, Surgeon Walter Coles, and Assistant Surgeon Augustus R. Taylor, who had received their medical degrees in 1857, 1860, and 1857, respectively.) Representative Henry C. Chambers of Mississippi claimed to have seen "long furloughs granted to comparatively well men, while they were denied to poor, decrepid creatures." Such complaints prompted a letter to a Richmond newspaper from "A Georgian," whose command of the subject and inside knowledge of the Medical Department suggested that he worked in the SGO. (Surgeon Francis Sorrel was the only SGO officer from Georgia.) Condemning the entire department on the basis of isolated complaints was puerile, argued the correspondent. Furthermore, the board was directed to act in the interest of patients and the service only, but "all kinds of pleas have been brought to bear on the Board of Examiners to give the constituents of some members of Congress furloughs or discharges. . . . Are Members of Congress ired because this 'Board of boys' decline to sign false certificates? It is a shame that such influence should be used." As for the assertion that well men received furloughs while feeble ones did not, the correspondent commented sarcastically, "as a Member of Congress says so, of course he is competent to judge more justly than a Medical Doctor, and further discussion is useless."[19]

Shortly following this exchange, a Senate committee appointed to investigate complaints about hospitals opined that furlough and discharge decisions should rest with hospital surgeons, who knew their patients best, rather than with the board. The committee noted, however, that the board's power was restricted in that it could grant a furlough only "if absolutely necessary to the recovery of the soldier's health." Legislation dealing with furloughs would not be passed and then approved by President Davis until May 1863, although the War Department extended the board system and repeatedly modified it during that time.[20]

On September 29, 1862, the AIGO issued General Orders No. 72, which directed that, outside of Richmond, a board of two or more medical officers would be established for each post or general hospital to examine soldiers for possible furlough or discharge. Board recommendations were to be approved by the hospital's senior surgeon and the commandant of the post. In December General Orders No. 107 specified that the aforementioned panels should grant furloughs only when the soldier's health required removal to another place or a change of climate. The orders added that boards could be suspended when the object of the pertinent paragraph of General Orders No. 72—to reduce the number of hospitalized patients—had, for the time being, been accomplished. This was an unusual acknowledgment that reducing a hospital's occupancy could be an object in itself. Doing so would have the practical benefits of providing beds for an influx of patients, lessening the workload in an understaffed hospital, or in an overcrowded facility, helping restore a healthier amount of space for each patient. In late April 1863 General Orders No. 51 summarized the pertinent procedures. For a soldier present with his regiment or company, his disability for military service would be attested to by his captain and the battalion or regimental surgeon, then the discharge documents would proceed up the chain of command for approval. A soldier with a temporary disability requiring a change of location could be granted a furlough of thirty days by the commander of his army or department. A hospitalized soldier away from his company, battalion, or regiment could be examined by a board of at least two medical officers for a thirty-day furlough, which required approval of the commandant of the post and was subject to extension.[21]

Officers found it difficult to understand the objects and operation of the furlough system. Surgeon Lafayette Guild, medical director of the Army of Northern Virginia, told Surgeon General Moore in January 1863, "Genl Lee is unwilling that the commander of another Department or Army should grant these privileges to officers and men of his army," a reference to soldiers of his command being treated in Richmond or at other places distant from his army. The same month, Guild tried to dispel a belief apparently held by Major General J. E. B. Stuart that patients were furloughed from general hospitals to make room for others. He denied that claim and held that, although they were "necessary for the efficiency of the army," the purpose of furloughs and discharges was to hasten recovery by "change of scene, mode of life &c." Guild may have been correct about their primary goal, but a House committee had acknowledged that beds vacated by furloughed soldiers "could be appropriated to other patients, thus greatly increasing the capacity of the hospitals to accommodate a greater number of patients in given time." Furthermore, when a great influx of new cases was expected in Richmond in June 1864, Medical Director of Hospitals Carrington encouraged Surgeon James B. McCaw at Chimborazo Hospital to have the examining board there grant furloughs or leaves of absence to all patients entitled to them.[22]

On May 1, 1863, President Davis approved new legislation that retained the board system. In places with three or more hospitals, a board of examiners would be created and consist of surgeons in charge of hospitals or of hospital divisions. The panel would visit the area hospitals, examine applicants for furlough or discharge, and grant furloughs for patients likely to be unfit for duty for at least thirty days; the furlough would be for the likely duration of disability up to sixty days, with no further approval necessary. Discharges recommended by the board required approval of the surgeon general or the commander of the army or department to which the soldier belonged. In locations with fewer than three hospitals, boards would be reduced in size accordingly. Furloughs were not to be granted if the members believed that "the life or convalescence of the patient would be endangered thereby." The act was put into operation at the end of May by AIGO General Orders No. 69, which noted that boards and post commandants could recommend but not grant leaves of absence to officers; such approval had to come from the commander of the army or department to which the officer belonged. Various modifications were made. One resulting from new legislation in February 1864 specified that the likely duration of disability needed for granting a furlough was now extended to be at least sixty (instead of thirty) days; the furlough would then be for sixty days.[23]

Surgeon Carrington noted problems with existing regulations in June 1864. He was expecting a large influx of wounded into Richmond hospitals and feared the consequences of overcrowding. Since the problem was likely to be temporary, a new act of Congress was unnecessary, but he asked that the secretary of war allow medical boards in Virginia's general hospitals to issue furloughs to men who were likely to be unfit for thirty days, instead of the sixty recently legislated, and to allow them to grant leaves of absence of the same length for officers, who were treated differently by General Orders No. 69. The various approvals for leaves of absence took so long to procure, said Carrington, that delays of a week or longer were common before a leave took effect. If patients who should be away on furlough or on leave remained hospitalized, the admission of large numbers of wounded soldiers would lead to "dangerous infectious diseases which will prove as fatal to slightly wounded as to the others." Finally, said Carrington to the surgeon general, "I am also informed by members of congress that the act [of May 1, 1863] regulating furloughs" and put into practice by General Orders No. 69 "was supposed to apply *to all sick and wounded officers and men*." In fact, the act, as worded, referred to "soldiers" and "furloughs," and legislators may not have realized that those terms—when applied by military men—did not encompass officers and leaves of absence.[24]

The condition that furloughs be denied if they were likely to endanger patients stemmed from surgeons' beliefs that soldiers were often more likely to recover if they remained hospitalized and received vigilant care than if they were sent home. Surgeon Carrington was "convinced that furloughs granted for 60 days frequently detain men from duty after they recover." Those thought ill enough to require such a long furlough, he noted, would "frequently recover sooner under better influences" in a hospital. Surgeon Guild cited cases in which men who had sustained wounds "of a trifling nature" developed "anchylosis [permanent fixation or stiffening of a joint], atrophy or contraction of the muscles and other deformities" when sent home. Furloughed soldiers were "out of reach of surgical aid. Their wounds are neglected, or the men themselves keep open their wounds or retain their limbs in abnormal positions during the process of healing, so that they never return to the army except as applicants for light duty or retirement." Guild suggested to General Lee that a properly constituted board of surgeons should recommend furlough or leave for patients whose wounds would eventually disable them from performing active service. Men with less serious wounds would be better off remaining in the care of surgeons for the above reasons. Guild's appeal suggests that furloughs and leaves in Lee's command were not granted in accordance to regulations or that boards under the general's influence were making decisions that were not in the best interest of the service.[25]

The Invalid Corps

The continuing need for soldiers and a desire to provide for disabled military personnel led to the formation of the Invalid Corps. According to legislation approved on February 17, 1864, and put into operation by AIGO general orders on March 16, men of the army and navy who were disabled in the line of duty by wounds or sickness could be retired or discharged from their previous position while retaining their rank, pay, and emoluments. The benefits of assignment to the Invalid Corps would continue for the duration of the war or until a recipient ceased to be retired or discharged. Disability would be certified by "one of the medical boards now established by law," and reexamination at least once every six months was required to document continued disability; recovery would result in restoration to duty. Applicants found incapable of full service in the field could be assigned or detailed to some appropriate duty, which could free some other soldier for service in the field. Because the relevant orders of the AIGO specified that the medical boards must comprise three medical officers, the apparent intent was that these would be the same panels already formed for determining eligibility for medical furlough, leave of absence, or discharge; conscription boards had, at most, two medical officers. Further legislation in January 1865 opened the Invalid Corps to disabled individuals, pending a medical examination, who had resigned their commission in ignorance of or before the formation of the corps. The 1865 legislation reduced the compensation of retired Invalid Corps officers to half pay, without other allowance or emoluments, unless they were assigned to duty.[26]

When Surgeon General Moore forwarded to the AIGO in early April 1864 the report of an examining board regarding applicants for the Invalid Corps, Cooper's office had to inquire what instructions he had given the panels. The efficient Moore had taken only eight days after the issuance of the AIGO's orders to provide detailed guidance to his medical directors. Cooper's staff was probably surprised by the speed with which the Medical Department's officers were submitting the required information.[27]

The War Department sought to ensure that men who were physically able to serve the military did so. At the same time, individuals had to be excluded or released if, because of disabilities, they would be a burden to the system. In cooperating to strike this balance, the Medical Department drew criticism when decisions made by its examining boards seemed inconsistent or unfair. Although the boards were convenient culprits, their actions were guided by the imperative to maximize the Confederacy's fighting force.

14. ❄ War's End and Beyond

The Confederate government fled Richmond on April 2, 1865, after General Robert E. Lee informed President Davis that he was unable to repel oncoming Union troops at Petersburg. As late as April 1, Surgeon General Moore was in the capital requesting the issuance of orders (regarding the assignment of medical officers) from the AIGO, also still in Richmond. The evacuation evidently included Moore, his fellow officers in the SGO, and other medical officers in staff positions. Their exact actions are unclear, however, and in most cases must be inferred from letters and parole and pardon documents.[1]

From Flight to Parole

The escape from Richmond of two groups is fairly well documented. One consisted of Jefferson Davis, most of his cabinet, and various other persons. The other comprised naval personnel escorting the so-called Confederate treasure—a large quantity of gold, silver, and bullion belonging to the government and some Richmond banks. Neither the surgeon general nor any other Medical Department personnel are mentioned in accounts of those escapes, and it is probable that Moore was in a separate group. He stopped (at least) at Charlotte, North Carolina; Newberry, South Carolina; and Augusta, Georgia, sites that were on the route of the treasure escort, but arrived at Charlotte two days before and at Augusta about a week after the treasure group. The routes of Moore and the Davis entourage appear to have overlapped for a day or two at Charlotte. According to a news story citing "the most reliable source," the surgeon general abandoned "the books, accounts, reports, and, in fact, all of the papers and important documents" of the SGO "during his hasty retreat from that town [Charlotte]." The article claimed that those records were captured. On the other hand, Moore said after the war that "nearly all the valuable documents of the [Medical] Department" were destroyed in the fire that consumed part of Richmond during the night of the evacuation and that "if any [documents] fell into the hands of the northern armies after we surrendered they were not of much importance." The whereabouts of the

Medical Department documents described in the news story, if they indeed survived the war, is unknown.[2]

On April 6 Moore, who had just arrived at Charlotte, telegraphed his location to Adjutant and Inspector General Cooper in Danville, Virginia. On April 19 Medical Purveyor J. J. Chisolm wrote multiple letters to him, one of which was addressed to the surgeon general in Charlotte. Chisolm was writing from Newberry, South Carolina, where he had moved supplies originally held at the medical-purveying depot in Columbia. That material had first been moved in February 1865 to Chester, South Carolina, just before Union troops occupied Columbia, then later to Newberry. On April 21 Moore, writing from Newberry, instructed Chisolm, also in Newberry, to send certain medical supplies to Augusta and to invoice them to Assistant Surgeon Edwin S. Ray, director of the medical-purveying depot there. On the twenty-fifth Moore, now in Augusta, directed Chisolm to turn over all of the Confederate money in his possession, minus an amount sufficient to pay his employees for the month, to a Mr. Wharton, who would convey the funds to Ray. The next day Moore informed Cooper that he had established his office in Augusta and asked for instructions. He also asked the general to give Surgeon James T. Johnson, director of the Charlotte medical-purveying depot, the authority to take actions—unspecified in this communication—with the medical supplies in his possession. That same day he ordered Chisolm to turn over all the government cotton in his possession to an authorized agent; Ray would receive payment for the cotton. Although Moore's letters said nothing about the purpose behind his orders, it seems likely that the surgeon general was organizing medical support for Confederate forces should they continue to fight. Chisolm's April 19 letters to him dealt with the movement of medical supplies and with the purveyor's plans to continue obtaining medical goods and rebuilding the distillery and medical laboratory in Columbia. By that time both were probably aware of the surrender on April 9 of the Army of Northern Virginia but acted as if the war would continue. General Joseph E. Johnston surrendered the troops under his command on April 26, an act that essentially ended the war east of the Mississippi.[3]

Available records do not indicate who accompanied Moore as he left Richmond. The handwriting on his April 21 letter and one of his April 26 letters, all above his signature, closely resembles that of Joseph F. Snipes, a conscript and corresponding clerk in the SGO whose services Moore considered indispensable. Moore was paroled in Augusta during May 1865 and signed a loyalty oath in Richmond on June 22. Thomas H. Williams, of the SGO staff, was paroled on May 9 in Augusta and signed a loyalty oath in Richmond on the same day as Moore; in fact, the oaths bore consecutive serial numbers. Thus, Williams may have accompanied Moore during the surgeon general's travels away from and then back to Richmond.[4]

Little is known about the end-of-war actions of Moore's other colleagues in the SGO. Charles H. Smith, his right-hand man in the office, was paroled at Greensboro, North Carolina, in late April. Francis Sorrel was paroled at Lynchburg, Virginia, on May 20, and Herman Baer was paroled at Appomattox Court House on April 9 as acting brigade surgeon of Gary's Brigade (cavalry). The only medical officer of the SGO remaining in Richmond as the war ended was Charles Brewer. At the time of the evacuation, he was relieved of his SGO duties and named "medical director of hospitals in charge of the sick and wounded" in the city; he was paroled in Richmond on April 18.[5]

Brewer's appointment allowed the departure from Richmond of William A. Carrington, who up to that time had been medical director of hospitals for Virginia. Carrington was paroled at Danville, Virginia, on April 28. The medical purveyor for Richmond, Edward W. Johns, was paroled at Greensboro, North Carolina, on May 1. Available records do not indicate what the SGO staff, Carrington, or Johns did or intended to do before their paroles.[6]

Postwar Activities of the Former Surgeons General

The former Confederate surgeons general led relatively quiet postwar lives. David Camden DeLeon settled in Mexico with other former Confederates. After a year there he relocated to New Mexico, where he had been stationed for several years when in the US Army and still owned some land. He worked there as a planter and physician until his death in 1872. According to an obituary, DeLeon's "last years were darkened by exile, disease and suffering—and death came to him as a deliverance." His recorded Civil War service was short, and there is too little known about it to judge his performance or influence on the Confederate Medical Department. DeLeon has been largely relegated to obscurity, with occasional mentions—often in publications about Jewish Americans (he was of Sephardic Jewish heritage)—emphasizing his Mexican War exploits.[7]

Charles H. Smith worked after the war in Richmond as a medical examiner for a life-insurance company and served as a board member of the Virginia Penitentiary. He died in 1879 while attending to business in Washington, DC. Practically nothing is known today about Smith's performance when temporarily in charge of the SGO, a position he held for several days only, or afterward as the de facto assistant surgeon general. But Smith's service in the SGO was praised early in the twentieth century when Confederate veterans were contemplating a monument commemorating Moore. "The Confederate hospital service," said a Richmond newspaper at the time, "was a wonderful institution.... What it was it was largely through the efforts of Moore and Charles H. Smith, his splendid assistant. The monument to the former should bear an inscription to the latter."[8]

As previously mentioned, Samuel Preston Moore was not pardoned for his part in the war until late 1866. He settled in Richmond, where he bought a house at 202 West Grace Street, next to the building he had occupied during the latter half of the war. Although he appeared in city directories as a physician, he did not establish a medical practice but instead participated in various organizations, such as the Virginia Agricultural Society—perhaps a reflection of his wartime interest in medicinal flora—and the Richmond School Board. He was elected a member of the R. E. Lee Camp of the Confederate Veterans of Richmond and first president of the Association of Medical Officers of the Confederate States Army and Navy, established in 1874. Moore's 1875 address at the second annual meeting of the last-mentioned organization appears to have been his only postwar account of his and his department's wartime activities. Moore died at his home on West Grace Street on May 31, 1889, and was buried in Richmond's Hollywood Cemetery.[9]

In 1909 the association of former Confederate medical officers adopted a resolution calling for a monument to Moore and the Medical Department to be erected in Richmond. The monument was never built, and the only known marker devoted to him is a stone tablet originally affixed to the house at 200 West Grace Street, where the surgeon general lived from the spring of 1863 until the end of the war. That tablet now appears on the Richmond Police Headquarters building, located at the same address at the northwest corner of West Grace and North Jefferson Streets. Histories touching on Civil War medical care have, evidently without exception, praised Moore's efficiency and effectiveness, but no full-length biography of Moore has been published.[10]

For the officers who directed the SGO, the postwar years were quiet compared with the busy lives they led as Confederate surgeons and as US medical officers before the Civil War. David Camden DeLeon, Charles H. Smith, and Samuel Preston Moore evidently left little in the form of journals or reminiscences than can help clarify the operations of the Confederate Medical Department and their personal contributions to the war effort. Surviving records, however, show that after its awkward formative months, the department became an admirable organization and a credit to the men who served in it.

✤ Conclusion

The Confederacy entered the Civil War unprepared for a long and severe conflict. It took the reasonable steps of modeling its government, including its War Department, after that of the United States and of giving responsible positions to officers who had recently been in the US Army. The tradition of seniority seemed to pay off in the assignment of Samuel Preston Moore to lead the Medical Department.

Moore's ability to shape his department as he wished, however, was limited. He was subordinate to President Davis—who constantly inserted himself into military affairs—and to the secretary of war, the latter office being filled by six men in succession over the course of the war. Moore also had another de facto superior, Adjutant and Inspector General Samuel Cooper, whose orders could be arbitrary and at odds with existing regulations. Although Congress demonstrated a general willingness to assist the Medical Department, it often failed to pass legislation that was helpful or could survive Davis's veto pen. Having multiple factions involved in creating regulations and policies sometimes resulted in confusing or contradictory orders.

Moore's efforts were often hampered by the inability of the Quartermaster and Subsistence Departments to provide the necessary assistance in erecting buildings or providing necessary supplies or food. Commanders' demands for fighting men threatened the Medical Department's workforce. The surgeon general had to fight for personnel and supplies meant for his department but desired by others.

Following tradition and precedent had its limitations, for the Confederate War Department quickly faced conditions that forced improvisation. Primary among those were the large size of the army and the inexperience of the men composing it. For the Medical Department, new organizational tiers had to be devised, and officers had to be assigned to head them. Although generals in the field tried to retain control of medical functions within their commands, the creation of medical directors of hospitals represented a movement of control away from those commanders and toward the surgeon general. Medical inspectors, originally tied to commands, also became responsible to the surgeon general only. Although the individual armies had their own medical purveyors, they generally obtained their supplies from depot purveyors, who also reported to the surgeon general and not to local commanders.

Shortages of medical supplies prompted Moore to initiate measures rather than simply purchase goods or supplies offered by blockade-runners. He worked with Confederate purchasing agents abroad and implemented a concerted effort to use indigenous plants. He ordered the establishment of medical laboratories to prepare indigenous and conventional medicines and, despite objections from governors, had his purveyors buy or operate distilleries for the production of medicinal alcohol. The surgeon general later assigned an officer to exchange cotton over enemy lines for medical supplies, a practice not uniformly approved by higher government officials.

Surgeon General Moore recommended a medical-evacuation system similar to that used by the French (and later by the Union) but was frustrated by the inability of Congress and President Davis to approve the necessary arrangements, by an inadequate number of medical officers, and by a constant shortage of ambulance wagons. As an alternative he resorted to creating the Reserve Surgical Corps to assist with care after major battles.

Under Moore's leadership, the army established a system of general hospitals that included some large facilities of the pavilion design favored by contemporary experts on the subject. In another move toward consolidation of control, he arranged for general hospitals originally operated by individual states to be closed or placed under Confederate government authority. During Moore's administration, specialty hospitals and wards were established for the care of patients with particular ailments, and dentists were assigned to visit general hospitals to treat patients in need of care. The Medical Department provided personnel and supplies for prison hospitals but could do little to improve conditions for POWs in or out of those facilities.

In the rush to build the army's strength, troops from the various states were quickly accepted into the Confederate service. Included with them were medical officers, some of whom proved unqualified. Surgeon General Moore quickly instituted medical examining boards to determine the fitness of surgeons already in the army, to review civilian applicants for appointment as medical officers, and to evaluate the merit of assistant surgeons applying for promotion to surgeon. Complaints about the examinations came from men who had already been appointed as medical officers and from applicants who thought the evaluations were unfair, yet the need for and general effectiveness of such screenings were confirmed by President Davis and the secretary of war. Knowing that illness often resulted from the failure of troops and their officers to observe basic sanitary practices, Moore encouraged the enforcement of relevant regulations and assigned inspectors to report on the cleanliness and management of medical facilities.

Moore placed high value on the collection, analysis, and dissemination of data. He thus ordered medical officers to regularly submit required reports and to inform his office of unusual patient cases. The SGO organized reports from the field and hospitals in hopes that lessons would emerge and contribute to patient care. Moore encouraged the publication of medical texts and a medical journal and helped organize an association of medical officers for the discussion of important clinical topics. He arranged for selected enlisted men to attend medical lectures so that they might become medical officers.

By assigning medical officers to examining boards and helping establish criteria for disability, the surgeon general assisted the War Department in excluding unfit men from the army and limiting the discharge of soldiers who were healthy enough to perform duty. Although Moore probably did not participate in decisions to declare fewer men unfit for duty, he certainly had a say in determining the specific medical criteria that the panels would use. He could not guarantee consistency of judgment among examining boards, and the need to maximize the army's fighting strength naturally made for unhappiness with some of their decisions.

The persistence and fighting ability of the Confederate military suggest that the Medical Department played a major role in maintaining the army's strength. Unfortunately, it is difficult to quantify the department's contribution or even to compare it with its counterpart in the Union army. The administrative core of the Confederate Medical Department comprised men who had recently served in the US Army, and the educational background of both Union and Confederate medical officers was probably similar. Thus, preferred procedures and treatments probably differed little between sides, and what medical officers were able to do depended largely on available resources. Compared with their Union counterparts, the Confederates were burdened with important disadvantages, including having fewer surgeons per regiment, fewer ambulance wagons, an unreliable supply chain, a less robust manufacturing base for producing medical goods, a smaller pool of nonphysician workers, a more rampant rate of inflation, a less reliable transportation system, and a homeland that was partially occupied or constantly threatened by the enemy. That Confederate soldiers received a lower quality of care would hardly be surprising, but even if that were to be proved—which it has not—the difference could not easily be attributed to factors within the control of the Medical Department.

Assessing the Medical Department's effectiveness might be facilitated by statistics that compared Union and Confederate sickness and death rates. The surviving data, however, are fragmentary and are neither particularly trustworthy nor directly comparable. The *Medical and Surgical History of the War of the Rebellion* summarized the information as follows: "So far as comparison can be made with the statistics at command, disease was not only more fatal among the Confederate forces, but the number of cases in proportion to the strength present was considerably greater among them than among the United States troops." Even with complete statistical reports, various factors other than the quality of care—differences between the sides in how cases were defined or recorded or in the baseline health or immunity of recruits, for example—could help explain such findings.[1]

Given the tradition of seniority and the officers available, it was probably inevitable that Moore would become the surgeon general of the Confederate army. That he would remain in that position was not guaranteed, so his service throughout the war may have indicated President Davis's general satisfaction with his performance. Moore's belief in military discipline seemed to serve him well in his post, but his dislike of politics and of pulling strings to get ahead may have made him an odd man out in Richmond. He also tended to micromanage, a trait possibly developed during his long duty as a US Army surgeon on the frontier, where he may have learned to be self-sufficient and trust only himself to see that tasks were performed properly.

Moore was, in fact, criticized as surgeon general for not delegating responsibility and for not using his influence to help enact legislation that would be favorable to the Medical Department. Maintaining a staff of capable officers around him, he clearly did delegate responsibility, even if he signed most communications leaving the SGO. Moore also communicated with members of Congress and encouraged the passage of various bills, but vetoes by President Davis seemed to convince him that trying to improve matters through legislation was largely futile.

Moore's curt manner and his refusal to grant special favors, even to politicians, may have created enemies in Congress and made them unwilling to support measures to assist the Medical Department. Although inadequacies of the department were mentioned in newspapers, the public perception of Moore seems generally to have been one of competence. Medical officers in a position to judge his performance generally regarded the surgeon general as lacking in amiability but having excellent organizational and administrative skills while treating subordinates strictly but fairly.

Moore's experiences in the US Army—which gave him firsthand knowledge of harsh military life and of the duties assigned to his subordinates in the Confederate Medical Department—probably contributed to his expecting a high level of selfless performance, even from men who had recently been civilians. Moore threatened and took disciplinary measures against medical personnel whose behavior disappointed him, but he was willing to consider explanations and reverse his original decisions. Misunderstandings sometimes stemmed from the surgeon general's terse communications and may have been avoided with the addition of a few words of explanation.

Although some observers were quick to condemn Moore's abrupt personality or find fault with individual surgeons or hospitals, there were relatively few criticisms of his major wartime decisions by anyone in a position to render an informed opinion. Surgeon Francis Peyre Porcher opined that Moore erred gravely in assigning skilled medical officers to positions of high responsibility, such as medical director or medical purveyor, when they might have been more useful caring for patients and teaching other surgeons how to do so. Moore, however, not only followed the military tradition of assigning experienced men to positions with administrative responsibility but also probably believed that having competent men in those stations would help ensure smoother operation of the entire department and provide a beneficial influence on a larger number of medical officers. Edwin S. Gaillard noted that the Medical Department's examination of indigenous remedies dashed the "lingering hope" that "the plants of each section of country [the South, in this instance] were all-sufficient for the eradication of diseases peculiar to that country." Such was not Moore's hope, for the surgeon general simply wanted useful substitutes for hard-to-obtain conventional drugs; with the exception of quinine for malaria, curative medicines were rare if not unknown. In light of knowledge available at the time, searching for usable indigenous remedies was entirely rational.[2]

Moore could have devoted more supplies and medical officers to the care of POWs, but the decisions that led to horrendous conditions in prison facilities were made by his superiors. He attempted to mitigate the situation—and claim some control over prison hospitals—by having the AIGO declare that those facilities and general hospitals were to be operated on the same footing. But any benefit to POWs by actions on his part would have been balanced by a reduction in the care of Confederate soldiers, and the government's priorities in that regard were clear. Moore's culpability, if any, in the mistreatment of

POWs was well below that of the Confederate president, secretary of war, and adjutant and inspector general.

Postwar reminiscences of the Confederate Medical Department and its leadership were laudatory, sometimes extremely so. Charles W. Chancellor, former chief surgeon of Major General George Pickett's division, left this account: "Touched by the wand of his [Surgeon General Moore's] wisdom and energy, the Medical Department of the Confederate Army sprang, Minerva like, prosperous and strong from his brain, and advanced with unfaltering steps to the front rank of all the departments, both in efficiency and organization and the high character of its officers." Perhaps more fitting—and more consistent with the tone of other assessments—was another of Chancellor's observations: "[Moore] accomplished phenomenal results considering the limited resources at his command." Former medical officer Samuel E. Lewis characterized the Medical Department's administration as demonstrating "marvellous discipline, efficiency and resourcefulness." Moore's obituary in Richmond's *Daily Dispatch* stated: "Many competent to judge have declared that the medical department was the best-managed department in the Confederacy. Certainly some of the disaster that befell our cause could have been averted had discipline as strict as he enforced everywhere prevailed." Porcher praised "the matchless organization of the medical department of the Confederate army as presented by the surgeon-general's office." (To be fair, the comparisons seemed to overlook the Ordnance Department—"one of the few bureaucratic bright spots in the Confederacy's dismally organized war effort"—and its commander, Josiah Gorgas.)[3]

Surgeon J. J. Chisolm, who had managed a medical-purveying district containing the Confederacy's busiest blockade-running ports, observed European military medical care, established a private hospital before the Civil War and a government one during it, and written a textbook for Confederate surgeons, was unusually well qualified to render an opinion about the Medical Department. In 1864, late enough for him to understand the progress of the war and the government bureaucracy but too early to be swept up in nostalgia, Chisolm praised Moore's efficiency in heading "the best organized of all the departments of our army." Comparisons aside, and in light of the conditions under which it operated, it is fair to characterize the Confederate Medical Department's performance as above any reasonable expectation and eminently worthy of study.[4]

Appendixes
Notes
Bibliography
Index

Appendix A
Selected Individuals in or Influencing the Confederate Medical Department

Baer, Herman. Medical officer and member of the SGO who compiled statistics.

Benjamin, Judah P. Second Confederate secretary of war (September 1861–March 1862).

Blackie, George S. Depot purveyor for northern Georgia and director of the medical laboratory at Atlanta (later Augusta).

Breckinridge, John C. Last (sixth) Confederate secretary of war (February–May 1865). Breckinridge had previous served as a major general in the Confederate army.

Brewer, Charles. Medical officer and member of the SGO. Brewer was left in charge of Richmond hospitals after the evacuation of the city in April 1865.

Carrington, William A. Medical director of hospitals for Virginia for the latter half of the war. Carrington had previously served as temporary medical director for the Department of North Carolina and Southern Virginia and was the corresponding secretary of ARMS.

Chisolm, J. J. Depot purveyor at Charleston and Columbia and director of the medical laboratory at Columbia. Chisolm wrote a textbook on military surgery and advised Surgeon General Moore about purveying concerns.

Cooper, Samuel. Adjutant and inspector general and highest-ranking officer in the Confederate army. Cooper was a confidant of President Davis and evidently bypassed the secretary of war in issuing orders affecting the Medical Department.

Covey, Edward N. Medical director of hospitals for North Carolina; removed from that post on request of that state's governor. Later, as a medical inspector, Covey urged that Medical Purveyor Potts be allowed to trade cotton for medical supplies and informed the surgeon general about the interdental split developed by dentist James Baxter Bean.

Davis, Jefferson. President of the Confederate States. Although Davis professed support for the Medical Department, he vetoed various bills intended to support it.

DeLeon, David Camden. First acting surgeon general of the Confederate army's Medical Department. DeLeon was relieved from that position and replaced by Charles Smith. He then served as medical director of the Department of Norfolk and the Army of Northern Virginia.

Gaillard, Edwin S. Medical director of various commands and an inspector. Gaillard developed a plan for medical evacuation and commented on a similar plan proposed by Surgeon General Moore. He had an arm amputated after being wounded during the Battle of Seven Pines.

Guild, Lafayette. Medical director of the Army of Northern Virginia for most of the war. Guild succeeded DeLeon in that position.

Huse, Caleb. Artillery officer who served in Europe purchasing ordnance and medical supplies.

Johns, Edward W. Depot purveyor at Richmond, director of the Richmond medical laboratory, and so-called chief purveyor for about a year. Johns served in the SGO before it moved from Montgomery to Richmond.

Lee, Robert E. Commanding general of the Army of Northern Virginia. Lee's interests sometimes conflicted with Surgeon General Moore's operation of the Medical Department.

McCaw, James Brown. Faculty member at MCV. McCaw helped develop Richmond's Chimborazo Hospital and, as a medical officer, served as its surgeon in charge. The *Confederate States Medical and Surgical Journal* reportedly operated under his charge. He also served as an ARMS director.

Miles, William Porcher. Chairman of the Committee on Military Affairs of the Provisional Congress and of the same House committee in the permanent Congress. Miles assisted in the drafting of legislation that would assist the Medical Department.

Moore, Samuel Preston. Surgeon general of the Confederate army's Medical Department for most of the Civil War. Moore succeeded DeLeon and Charles Smith in that office.

Myers, Abraham C. Quartermaster general for the first half of the war. Myers's department was often blamed for shortcomings in supporting the Medical Department.

Northrop, Lucius B. Commissary general until early 1865. Northrop evidently agreed that Union POWs would have lower priority in receiving rations than Confederate soldiers.

Porcher, Francis Peyre. Medical officer and botanist best known for writing *Resources of the Southern Fields and Forests* at the direction of Surgeon General Moore.

Potts, Richard. Medical director for the Western Department early in the war and depot purveyor for Mississippi, western Tennessee, and Arkansas. Potts was assigned by Surgeon General Moore to take charge of exchanging cotton over enemy lines for medical supplies.

Prioleau, William H. Depot purveyor at Savannah and Macon and director of the medical laboratory at Macon.

Randolph, George W. Third Confederate secretary of war (March–November 1862). Randolph had previously been an army officer serving in Virginia.

Seddon, James. Fifth Confederate secretary of war (November 1862–February 1865).

Smith, Charles Henry. Temporary surgeon general of the Confederate army's Medical Department after DeLeon was relieved. Smith continued in the SGO under Moore as the de facto assistant surgeon general.

Smith, Gustavus Woodson. Interim (fourth) Confederate secretary of war for a few days in November 1862. Smith, a major general, commanded the Department of North Carolina and Southern Virginia, which included the defenses of Richmond.

Sorrel, Francis. Medical inspector of hospitals and member of the SGO. Sorrel compiled statistics regarding the sick and wounded and stated that he helped establish general hospitals east of the Mississippi River.

Stout, Samuel H. Superintendent of hospitals and later medical director of hospitals for the Army of Tennessee.

Walker, Leroy Pope. First Confederate secretary of war (February–September 1861).

Williams, Thomas Henry. Medical director of the Army of Northern Virginia, replaced in that position by DeLeon. Williams became part of the SGO in charge of medical purveying.

Winder, John. Inspector general of military camps around Richmond, then commander of the post at Andersonville and commissary general of prisoners. Winder was named, after his death, as a coconspirator in the trial of Wirz.

Wirz, Henry. Commander of the prison stockade at Andersonville. Wirz was executed after being convicted of war crimes in a trial that implicated former surgeon general Moore as a coconspirator.

Appendix B
Staff of the Surgeon General's Office, November 1864

Military Officers

Surgeon Samuel Preston Moore, age 49, appointed from South Carolina: Surgeon General.

Surgeon Charles Henry Smith, age 45, appointed from Virginia: Acting Assistant Surgeon General (services absolutely indispensable).

Surgeon Thomas Henry Williams, age 35, appointed from Texas: Assistant in charge of purveying business of the Medical Bureau (services absolutely indispensable).

Surgeon Francis Sorrel, age 37, appointed from Georgia: Assistant in charge of reports and records of sick and wounded, and inspector of hospitals in Richmond (services absolutely indispensable).

Surgeon Charles Brewer, age 32, appointed from Maryland: Assistant specially in charge of records of conscription, examining validity of exemptions, and general business of the office (services absolutely indispensable).

Surgeon Herman Baer, age 34, appointed from South Carolina: Assistant in tabulating and arranging statistics of reports of sick and wounded, certificates for retirement, and examining inspection reports (services absolutely indispensable).

Civilian Clerks

J. T. Newberry, age 35, from Georgia: Chief clerk (services absolutely indispensable).

George C. Wedderburn, age 25, from Louisiana, unfit for field service: General business of the office (services indispensable).

Information and remarks are as indicated in Return of Civil and Military Officers, file 3055, entry 183, RG 109. Names were completed or corrected on the basis of listings and signatures in other records (87-IV-RG109; 88-IX-RG109; files 3090, 3176, 3680, 4748, entry 60, RG 109; and files 4451, 4780, 5020, 5114, 5310, 5332, entry 183, RG 109).

Russell S. Betts, age 26, from Virginia, unfit for field service: Records of medical officers (services necessary).

George T. Turner, age 30, from Georgia, unfit for field service: Hospital accounts (services necessary).

Thomas I. E. Fox, age 28, from Maryland, disabled: Records, letters referred, and appointments of hospital stewards (services necessary).

Joseph C. Meador, age 45, from Virginia: Property accounts of medical officers (services necessary).

Harry C. Morris, age 28, druggist, from North Carolina: In charge of examinations of medical officers and returns of public property (services indispensable).

Theodore T. White, age 31, from Georgia, disabled: Assistant for medical officers' records (services necessary).

Men Detailed for Clerical Duty

Joseph F. Snipes, age 20, conscript, appointed from Virginia: Corresponding clerk (services indispensable).

L. B. Edwards, age 19, private, appointed from Virginia: Examining inspection reports (services necessary).

W. C. Schwalmyer, age 27, conscript, appointed from Virginia, disabled: Examining medical purveyors' accounts (services necessary).

A. G. Baylor, age 29, hospital steward, appointed from Virginia, disabled: Mail and records of conscription (services necessary).

R. Dykers, age 26, hospital steward, appointed from Louisiana, unfit for field service: In charge of files of the office (services necessary).

M. Clark, age 32, hospital steward, appointed from Georgia: Examining medical purveyors' accounts (services necessary).

R. Axson, age 27, hospital steward, appointed from Louisiana: Examining medical purveyors' accounts (services necessary).

J. Cary Jordan, age 28, hospital steward, appointed from Virginia, disabled: Examining inspectors' reports (services necessary).

A. S. Thomson, age 25, hospital steward, appointed from Virginia, disabled: Corresponding, purveyors' letters and endorsements (services indispensable).

H. S. Breeden, age 27, private, state not indicated, disabled: Examining inspectors' reports (services necessary).

J. Marshall Caldwell, age 28, hospital steward, appointed from South Carolina, disabled: Endorsements (services necessary).

Female Clerks

L. G. Winn: Examining hospital fund accounts (services necessary).

Lizzie Page Nelson: Examining medical officers' accounts (services necessary).

B. S. Saunders: Examining hospital fund accounts (services necessary).

E. O. Beall: Copying letters from office (services necessary).

Maria P. Steger: Copying references of official letters (services necessary).

Fannie G. Halyburton: Examining medical officers' accounts (services necessary).

Grace F. McGuire: Examining medical officers' accounts (services necessary).

Julia Peyton: Endorsement clerk (services necessary).

J. Triplett: Examining medical officers' accounts (services necessary).

R. Macmurdo: Examining hospital fund accounts (services necessary).

Appendix C
Surgeon General Moore's Proposal for
a Medical Evacuation System

Sir:

Much of the difficulty and embarrassment heretofore experienced in securing to our armies in the field, the full efficiency of the Medical Department may be ascribed in part at least to its defective and imperfect organization; but it is more particularly in connection with the omission on the part of the framers of the laws creating and organizing the Medical Staff, to provide for supernumerary, or other than Regimental Medical Officers, that I am induced to submit for your consideration a plan for Field Ambulance or Provisional Hospitals.

It is true that by a law passed during the third session of the Confederate Congress, every possible latitude was granted to the Department for the appointment of Hospital Surgeons; but this clearly related to fixed or permanent Hospitals. In time of War it becomes absolutely necessary that supernumerary medical officers (so to speak) should accompany troops, the number to be regulated of course by the strength of the command, and the nature of the expedition. The moment an Army takes the field it finds itself separated from its Hospitals in the rear, and to obviate the difficulties, and inconveniences of at once transporting thence its sick and wounded Provisional or temporary Hospitals should be established nearby with suitable material and a sufficient "personnel." These can be made to follow if necessary, the marches, and counter-marches of an Army, its advances and retreats. The influence such a measure exerts on the success of military operations cannot be doubted; by being thus enabled to retain the sick, near the Regiments, and Corps the cured are sooner returned to duty and the maximum strength of the Army more perfectly maintained; while on the other

---

Copy, Samuel Preston Moore to William Porcher Miles, Chairman of the Committee on Military Affairs, Provisional Congress of the Confederate States, December 14, 1861, entry UD 176A, RG 109.

hand if they are altogether detached, and removed to remote points in the interior experience proves they need never again be counted on for the remainder of the campaign. But it is more especially during and after an engagement that this class of officers become really invaluable and almost indispensable to the security and comfort, nay even the recovery oftentimes of so many of the wounded, for then the Regimental Surgeons are not in sufficient force to attend to all and but for their aid, and presence, numbers must lie for hours neglected with undressed, stiff, and painful wounds.

The following description of the proposed plan of operations as derived from and now in use by the French, may serve perhaps to illustrate more forcibly its nature and character, and to afford evidence of its usefulness at such times.

As soon as an "Affair" is about to begin the Ambulance, or Hospital Depots are established slightly to the rear of the lines, and beyond the range of projectiles—if all together under the immediate charge of the Medical Director, but if scattered according to their respective Brigades, then under the direction of their respective Brigade Surgeons.

The spot, or spots should be chosen when practicable in villages, farm houses, or barns, but in every case so that free communication may be had with the front which is in action, and with the rear, whence is to be derived the Ambulance wagons necessary to transport the wounded to a distance from the theatre of war, after the proper dressings have been supplied.

An Order of the day usually indicates to the different corps the exact positions of the ambulances to which should be sent their respective wounded. The first disposition being now made, a number of ambulance officers mounted on spring wagons, and provided with *litters*, lint dressings, instruments, and a few of the more necessary medicines, such as stimulants &c, repair together with the *soldier nurses*, to the field succor there such of the wounded, as are retained on the spot, and to send them, as *quickly as possible*, on litters in spring wagons to the nearest depot.

When the number of wounded sent to the different ambulance depots is very considerable, a number of the staff Surgeons heretofore engaged in lending aid in the field, return to the depots of their respective Brigades or Divisions, where under the supervision of their respective Chiefs all are engaged with their appropriate duties, the younger and less experienced extract bullets superficially located, bandage and dress simple flesh wounds, while the older and more skillful perform operations, amputate, and reduce fractures, and apply apparatus. The Regimental Medical Officers, too at this time repair with a similar object to the depots of their respective regiments, and assist in the same way.

And now those slightly wounded, in the upper extremities, but not able to be returned to their regiments, are marched to some neighboring Hospital while others, more seriously affected, such as amputations, penetrating wounds of the chest, head, or abdomen, or fractures are placed on litters in spring wagons, brought up for that purpose from the rear, and sent to the same destinations; to accompany these latter and attend to their wants in transit one or more of the *ambulance Surgeons*, should be detailed. This movement continued regularly from the line of battle to the ambulance depot, and thence to the Hospitals, or railroad termini in the rear, will if regularly maintained without confusion and crowding, enable the wounded to be quickly, and comfortably removed from the field.

When finally the field Infirmaries are no longer supplied with fresh cases, they break up, and disperse, each Brigade with the exception of such of the ambulance officers, and nurses, as may have been detailed to remain with, or accompany the sick, assembles at its own Head Quarters, the personnel, and material belonging to it.

Such is a brief and imperfect sketch of the plan now in use by the French, and which I desire to see in part at least adopted into our service.

It will be observed that each Brigade in keeping separate and distinct its Ambulance organization can be in readiness at any moment to undertake service, detached and at a distance from the main body of an Army, and yet when together with other Brigades these may be temporarily coalesced to render more efficiently the service expected of them. It will be observed also, in this system that there need never be any occasion for detaching *regimental* Medical Officers from the legitimate sphere of their duties. Should it be necessary in the ordinary advance and forward movements of an Army to send to the rear its sick, they fall at once into the hands of the Staff Surgeons, and are properly cared for.

In the event of casualties or sickness among the same class of officers a supernumerary, or staff Surgeon, is ready on the spot to be assigned to duty as such, and thus Regiments can always enjoy the presence of the authorized number of medical officers.

To accomplish this object, then it will only be necessary for Congress to pass a law, creating a certain number of Staff Surgeons, and Staff Asst. Surgeons, and also a corps of soldier or Military Nurses. The duties of these latter as may be inferred from previous allusions will consist alike in rendering aid on the battle field, in supplying litters, lint dressing, and in assisting the wounded to the depots, or Field Infirmaries, and at other times, both before, and after battle as ordinary Apothecaries, and Nurses in Hospital.

They should be designated by some particular uniform, so that there will be no difficulty in recognizing them, any where, and should only be armed for personal protection, against stragglers with Colts Revolvers. Their presence during a battle will obviate much of the embarrassment so commonly provoked by the "falling out of ranks" of soldiers for the purpose, both real and imaginary of assisting their wounded comrades to the rear.

The material consisting of wagons, tents, litters, &c &c, can all be procured by existing regulations.

The accompanying sketch of a Bill, which tho' it may be imperfect in language, and form will serve to convey to you the idea of what I seek to accomplish, by enactment.

Trusting that you will give the subject your earnest attention

I remain Sir, With high respect, Your Obt. Servt.
(Signed) S. P. Moore, Surg. Gen'l

Notes

*All sources with a record group (RG) designator are from the Washing-
ton, DC, branch of the National Archives and Records Administration
(NARA). Most textual records from RG 109 are divided into chapters
indicated by roman numerals. RG 109 citations with a chapter designator
are shown in abbreviated form, with volume (and part, if applicable, in
parentheses) followed by chapter and "RG109." Thus, 741(1)-VI-RG109
represents volume 741, part 1, chapter VI, RG 109, NARA. Unless otherwise indicated, all microfilm is from RG 109. Roll numbers appear in
parentheses after the film identifier, so that microfilm M346(24) indicates
microfilm M346, roll 24, RG 109, NARA. Unless otherwise indicated,
General Orders (GO) and Special Orders (SO) are from the Confederate Adjutant and Inspector General's Office (AIGO). Parentheses enclose
paragraph numbers, so that SO 80(1) indicates Special Orders No. 80,
paragraph 1. The* Journal of the Congress of the Confederate States
of America, 1861–1865, *is abbreviated as* JCCSA. The War of the
Rebellion: A Compilation of the Official Records of the Union and
Confederate Armies *is abbreviated as* OR.

Introduction

1. Act of Feb. 9, 1861, chap. 1, Prov. Cong. C.S.A. Stat. 27; War Department (Confederate), *Army Regulations*.
2. Butler, *Judah P. Benjamin*, 233–35.

1. Medical Department for a New Nation

1. Act of Feb. 26, 1861, chap. 17, Prov. Cong. C.S.A. Stat. 38; Cooper to Leroy Walker, Apr. 25, 1861, *OR*, ser. 4, 1:252–53; Act of May 16, 1861, chap. 20, § 4, Prov. Cong. C.S.A. Stat. 114, 115. Surgeons in the US Army had histor- ically been considered civil rather than line officers and were thus allowed an assimilated rather than actual rank. The assimilated rank corresponded to an actual rank for the purposes of ceremonies, protocol, and the like. Medical officers in the regular US Army were granted actual rank in 1847. Gillett, *Army Medical Department*, 129; Act of Feb. 11, 1847, chap. 8, § 9, 9 Stat. 123, 124–25.

2. Act of Mar. 6, 1861, chap. 26, § 9, Prov. Cong. C.S.A. Stat. 45, 46; Act of Aug. 14, 1862, chap. 21, Prov. Cong. C.S.A. Stat. 176; Gaillard, "Medical and Surgical Lessons," 716–17; "Medical Purveyors—The Rank of Surgeons," *Daily Richmond Examiner*, Apr. 13, 1863; "Medical Purveyors," *Daily Richmond Enquirer*, Apr. 15, 1863.

3. Davis, *Rise and Fall of the Confederate Government*, 1:309–10; Act of Mar. 14, 1861, chap. 41, § 5, Prov. Cong. C.S.A. Stat. 61, 62; Act of Feb. 26, 1861, chap. 17, Prov. Cong. C.S.A. Stat. 38.

4. *Official Army Register, for 1861*, 5–7; *Official Army Register, for 1862*, 75, 79; Surgeons and Assistant Surgeons, 88-I-RG109. Two US medical officers— Rodney Glisan and Aquila T. Ridgely—evidently resigned with no intent of serving the Confederacy, while a third, William J. L'Engle, died before achieving his wish to serve. Declaration of Madeleine M. L'Engle, file for L'Engle, microfilm M346(582).

5. Surgeons and Assistant Surgeons, 88-I-RG109; Moore to Andrew Johnson, June 23, 1865, microfilm M1003(65), RG 94. Thomas C. Madison resigned his position of full surgeon in the US Army on August 17, 1861, so he was not appointed surgeon in the regular Confederate army until November 1861.

6. SO 44(7), May 6, 1861, 6-I-RG109; Surgeons and Assistant Surgeons, 88-I-RG109. It is unclear whether William A. Carswell, formerly of the US Army, was appointed to the regular Confederate army or just to the PACS. DeLeon to Leroy Walker, Apr. 5, 1861, file 269, microfilm M437(1). Also unclear is whether it became automatic for assistant surgeons in the regular army to be appointed full surgeons in the PACS. Andrew J. Foard and Robert L. Brodie, assistant surgeons in the regular army, each received his appointment as surgeon, PACS, after asking for it. Brodie complained that such appointments had already been granted to medical officers who had been junior to him in the US Army. Foard to Samuel Cooper, Aug. 17, 1861, with endorsements, microfilm M331(95); Brodie to Leroy P. Walker, Aug. 30, 1861, microfilm M331(34).

7. *Official Army Register, for 1861*, 5; "Death of a South Carolinian Abroad," *Charleston (SC) Daily News*, Sept. 25, 1872, 1; Wiernik, *History of the Jews in America*, 162; DeLeon to Thomas Lawson, Mar. 21, 1860, file D43, microfilm M567(622), RG 94.

8. DeLeon to Samuel Cooper, Feb. 19, 1861, file D46, microfilm M619(15), RG 94; Woodward and Muhlenfeld, *Private Mary Chesnut*, 14; file for DeLeon, microfilm M331(74); SO 32(6), Apr. 22, 1861, 6-I-RG109; SO 44(7), May 6, 1861, ibid.; *JCCSA*, 1:50; Capers, *Life and Times of C. G. Memminger*, 330; City Hotel, advertisement, *Montgomery (AL) Daily Post*, July 4, 1865;

"The War in America," *Times* (London), May 30, 1861; DeLeon, *Four Years in Rebel Capitals*, 37.

9. Woodward and Muhlenfeld, *Private Mary Chesnut*, 17; Dauber, "David Camden DeLeon," 2929; DeLeon, *Four Years in Rebel Capitals*, 28; Moore to AIGO, May 13, 1861, 45-I-RG109. Moore's communication is described briefly in a register, but the entire letter has not been located. In Medical Department titles, the most common use of the word "acting" was in "acting assistant surgeon," which usually (but not always) referred to a civilian contract surgeon.

10. SO 59(3), May 25, 1861, and SO 64(2), June 5, 1861, 6-I-RG109; Jones, *Rebel War Clerk's Diary*, 1:32–33, 42; Vanfelson, *Little Red Book*, 9; "In Memoriam"; Crist, Williams, and Dillard, *Papers of Jefferson Davis*, 182n3; 1860 US Census, Montgomery County, AL, population schedule, 1st division, 60, dwelling 549, family 537, Wm. C. Ducksbry.

11. Holloway, "Reminiscences."

12. Samuel Cooper to DeLeon, May 1, 1861, 35-I-RG109; DeLeon to Cooper, June 5 (file 1246), June 12 (file 2138), and July 1, 1861 (file 2031), microfilm M437(3–5); DeLeon, *Four Years in Rebel Capitals*, 111–14.

13. SO 95(3), July 12, 1861, 6-I-RG109; DeLeon to Davis, July 12, 1861, and DeLeon to Smith, July 13, 1861, file 2727, microfilm M437(6); Walker to DeLeon, July 19, 1861, microfilm M522(1); DeLeon to Walker, July 20, 1861, file 2416, microfilm M437(5). Exactly which Virginia troops DeLeon supposedly failed to supply is unclear. Reports from Harpers Ferry and Laurel Hill, Virginia, in late May and late June 1861, respectively, indicated deficiencies in medical supplies. George Deas to Robert S. Garnett, May 23, 1861, *OR*, ser. 1, 2:867–70; Garnett to Deas, June 26, 1861, ibid., 236–38.

14. DeLeon to Walker, July 17, 1861, file 2357, microfilm M437(5); DeLeon to Walker, July 22, 1861, microfilm M331(74); DeLeon to AIGO, July 24, 1861, 45-I-RG109; Samuel Cooper to DeLeon, July 22, 1861, 35-I-RG109; DeLeon to AIGO, July 31, 1861, 46-I-RG109.

15. "The Whereabouts of Beauregard," *Charleston (SC) Mercury*, July 31, 1861.

16. SO 127(15), June 3, 1862, and SO 148(2), June 27, 1862, 9-I-RG109; Newton, "My Recollections," 486; Warren, *Doctor's Experiences*, 295–97; DeLeon to George W. Randolph, July 1862, microfilm M331(74); "Death of a South Carolinian Abroad," *Charleston (SC) Daily News*, Sept. 25, 1872; Johnson, *Twentieth Century Biographical Dictionary*, s.v. "De Leon, David Camden"; P. DeLeon, "Military Record of the DeLeon Family," 332; James Hunter Berrien to Edward P. Turner, July 10, 1863, file for Berrien, microfilm M331(23). In Berrien's letter, all persons other than DeLeon were referred to by a

military rank, so Berrien's use of "Dr." rather than "Surgeon" DeLeon may suggest that DeLeon was acting in a civilian capacity, perhaps as a contract surgeon. Whether David Camden DeLeon was meant, however, is unknown.

17. Woodward and Muhlenfeld, *Private Mary Chesnut*, 106, 107; "Local Matters," *Daily Dispatch* (Richmond), July 27, 1861; SO 110(9), July 30, 1861, 6-I-RG109; *Official Army Register, for 1861*, 5; Newton, "My Recollections," 486; "Death of a South Carolinian Abroad," *Charleston (SC) Daily News*, Sept. 25, 1872; *JCCSA*, 1:567–6 8, 844, 849; Surgeons and Assistant Surgeons, 88-I-RG109.

18. Farr, "Samuel Preston Moore"; *Official Army Register, for 1861*, 5; Payne, "Samuel Preston Moore's Letters"; Thomas Lawson to John B. Floyd, Feb. 28, 1859, file S67, microfilm M567(612), RG 94; "Obituary Record: Dr. Samuel Preston Moore."

19. Robert C. Wood to Samuel Cooper, Jan. 30, 1860, file for Wood, microfilm M567(632), RG 94; M. Grivot to Moore and Moore to Grivot, Jan. 28, 1861, *OR*, ser. 1, 1:497; DeLeon to Leroy P. Walker, Apr. 8, 1861, *OR*, ser. 4, 1:212; Moore to Lawson, Feb. 12, 1861, microfilm M619(36), RG 94; Webb to Davis, Feb. 20, 1861, microfilm M331(181).

20. Moore to Andrew Johnson, June 23, 1865, microfilm M1003(65), RG 94; Leroy P. Walker to Moore, Mar. 26, 1861, 119-I-RG109; Lewis, "Samuel Preston Moore," 383; *JCCSA*, 1:567–68.

21. Davis, "General Samuel Cooper"; Cooper appointment, Aug. 31, 1861, 119-I-RG109; Wilson, *Confederate Industry*, 87–88; Felt, "Lucius B. Northrop"; Northrop appointment, Nov. 26, 1864, 128-I-RG109; Vandiver, *Rebel Brass*, 23–27, 84.

22. War Department (Confederate), *Regulations for the Medical Department* (1861), 3; Bartholomees, *Buff Facings and Gilt Buttons*, 71.

23. Smith to Davis, Dec. 17, 1861, with Davis endorsement, file 8587, microfilm M437(18); Act of Feb. 26, 1861, chap. 17, § 6, Prov. Cong. C.S.A. Stat. 38, 39.

24. *JCCSA*, 5:288–89, 384, 454, 486–87, 493; ibid., 2:379, 380–81, 405–6, 415; "An Act to reorganize and promote the efficiency of the Medical Department of the Army," 1862, Internet Archive, https://archive.org/details /acttoreorganizep00conf (accessed Mar. 7, 2017).

25. Davis, veto message, Oct. 13, 1863, *JCCSA*, 5:557–58.

26. Yearns, *Confederate Congress*, 111; Coulter, *Confederate States of America*, 147; Cleland, "Jefferson Davis and the Confederate Congress," 221; Cunningham, "Organization and Administration," 389.

2. The Surgeon General and His Office

1. "The Mechanics Institute," *Richmond Enquirer*, Nov. 16, 1858; Moore to AIGO, Sept. 18, 1861, 46-I-RG109; Benjamin to Abraham Myers, Lucius Northrop, Josiah Gorgas, Moore, and Danville Leadbetter, Nov. 12, 1861, microfilm M522(3). The Mechanics Institute building was "surmounted by a large and conspicuous observatory." *Stranger's Guide*, 3. The difficult-to-impress Thomas Cooper DeLeon called the structure "an ungainly pile of bricks." DeLeon, *Four Years in Rebel Capitals*, 87.

2. Vanfelson, *Little Red Book*, 9, 17–18; *City Intelligencer*, 18; Cunningham, "Organization and Administration," 393; Act of Mar. 7, 1861, chap. 30, § 1, Prov. Cong. C.S.A. Stat. 52; Payrolls, 87-IX-RG109, 88-IX-RG109; Payrolls, files 3090, 3176, 3680, 4748, entry 60, RG 109; Misc. manuscripts, files 3055, 4451, 4780, 5020, 5114, 5310, 5332, entry 183, RG 109.

3. *Official Army Register, for 1861*, 6; Thomas Lawson to John B. Floyd, Oct. 5, 1860, letter S334, microfilm M567(633), RG 94; Newton, "My Recollections," 486; Vanfelson, *Little Red Book*, 9; *Stranger's Guide*, 11; "Government of the Confederate States: War Department," *Daily Chattanooga Rebel*, Jan. 7, 1865; Return of Civil and Military Officers, file 3055, entry 183, RG 109.

4. *Official Army Register, for 1861*, 7; Brewer to Andrew Johnson, May 11, 1865, microfilm M1003(57), RG 94; Return of Civil and Military Officers, file 3055, entry 183, RG 109; *Biographical Review*, 427–34; Moore to James A. Seddon, Dec. 13, 1864, file H-570, microfilm M437(130); John Withers, diary, June 1, 1862, entry 187, RG 109; "The Hospitals," *Richmond Whig and Public Advertiser*, June 3, 1862. One newspaper reported that a surgeon other than Peticolas performed the amputation. See "Amputated," *Daily Dispatch* (Richmond), June 3, 1862.

5. "Died," *Daily Dispatch* (Richmond), Oct. 21, 1862; *Biographical Review*, 427–34; Collins, *Collins Family*, 162; "The Death and Burial of Major-General J. E. B. Stuart, Flower of Cavaliers," *Daily Richmond Examiner*, May 14, 1864; *Year Book, 1909–1910*, 31.

6. Newton, "My Recollections," 484; *Official Army Register, for 1856*, 6; Mackall, "Late Doctor Francis Sorrel"; Sorrel, *Recollections*, 58; Return of Civil and Military Officers, file 3055, entry 183, RG 109. Robert L. Brodie, an assistant surgeon in the regular Confederate army, evidently believed that he had served in the US Army for a longer duration than Sorrel and should thus have been appointed surgeon before him. Secretary of War Seddon acknowledged Brodie's claim but said that Sorrel's appointment could not be undone. Seddon to J. Chesnut Jr., Feb. 7, 1863, microfilm M522(6).

7. Return of Civil and Military Officers, file 3055, entry 183, RG 109; *Official Army Register, for 1861*, 6; Williams to Abraham Lincoln, May 31, 1861, file W470, microfilm M619(67), RG 94; Williams to Andrew Johnson, July 12, 1865, microfilm M1003(30), ibid.; SO 130(6), June 6, 1862, 9-I-RG109; SO 293(16), Dec. 15, 1862, 11-I-RG109; SO 10(6), Jan. 13, 1863, and SO 11(24), Jan. 14, 1863, 207-I-RG109; Return of Civil and Military Officers, file 3055, entry 183, RG 109.

8. "Necrology: Herman Baer"; "Medical College of the State of South Carolina," *Charleston (SC) Mercury*, Mar. 12, 1861; Compiled service record (CSR) for Baer, file for Bair [*sic*], microfilm M331(12); Return of Civil and Military Officers, file 3055, entry 183, RG 109.

9. Return of Civil and Military Officers, file 3055, entry 183, RG 109; Sorrel, *Recollections*, 58.

10. Return of Civil and Military Officers, file 3055, entry 183, RG 109; Tower, *Lee's Adjutant*, 96, 272n45; Moore to Cooper, Nov. 21, 1864, file S3337, microfilm M474(145); Morris to George S. Barnsley, Oct. 27, 1863, *George Scarborough Barnsley Papers*; Moore to Cooper, Oct. 31, 1864, with endorsements, file M4052, microfilm M474(131). The handwriting of Moore's request to Cooper for Morris, dated October 31, 1864, which the surgeon general signed, matches that of Morris, who was on leave in Richmond at the time. Pay receipt, Jan. 1864, manuscript 5020, entry 183, RG 109.

11. Brock, *Richmond during the War*, 162–63; Sites to George S. Barnsley, June 5, Sept. 6, 1863, *George Scarborough Barnsley Papers*.

12. "Proceedings of the Association," 414; Jones, "Medical Corps," 347–50; Roberts, "Organization and Personnel," 349; Van Riper and Scheiber, "Confederate Civil Service," 459. Hambrecht and Koste's unpublished and privately maintained "Biographical Register of Physicians Who Served the Confederacy in Medical Capacity" has been compiled from Confederate documents (primarily CSRs) and other sources. The figures provided here were extracted by Hambrecht on July 6, 2019.

13. "Surg. Gen. Samuel Preston Moore," *Southern Illustrated News* (Richmond), Nov. 7, 1863.

14. Claiborne, *Seventy-Five Years in Old Virginia*, 198–200; Gholson, "Recollections," 36–37; Porcher to Virginia Porcher, Mar. 10, 15, 1862, Francis Peyre Porcher Papers, Waring Historical Library.

15. Moore to Carrington, Apr. 6, 1863, 740(1)-VI-RG109.

16. Surgeon General's Office, circulars, Sept. 30, Oct. 8, 1861, Jan. 4, 1862, 739(1)-VI-RG109; Williams to Moore, Nov. 23, 1861, 367-VI-RG109.

17. Moore to Randolph, May 21, 1862, file S1041, microfilm M474(47); GO 43(5), June 13, 1862, 2-I-RG109.

18. Moore to Carrington, July 21, 1863, file S1671, microfilm M474(83).

19. Porcher, "Confederate Surgeons," 15–16; Claiborne, *Seventy-Five Years in Old Virginia*, 199–200; Brock, *Richmond during the War*, 161–63; "City Alms House," *Daily Richmond Examiner*, Feb. 10, 1863; Long Grabs [Murdoch John McSween], untitled correspondence, *Fayetteville (NC) Observer*, Mar. 2, 1863.

20. Moore to McCaw, July 15, 1863, and McCaw to Moore, July 16, 1863, file for McCaw, microfilm M331(168); Moore to John C. Breckinridge, Feb. 9, 1865, *OR*, ser. 4, 3:1073–76; Moore to William Little, Mar. 25, 1864, Documenting the American South, https://docsouth.unc.edu/imls/medproperty/image.html. The hospital fund consisted of the value of rations allotted to but not used by patients. The fund could be used to purchase items, such as food delicacies, not typically obtained through the usual government supply chain.

21. Holloway, "Reminiscences."

22. Moore endorsement, Mar. 21, 1863, on Blackie receipt, Mar. 2, 1863, 750-VI-RG109.

23. Stephen A. Dodge to Randolph, June 21, 1862, with endorsements, *OR*, ser. 2, 4:782–83; Crocker, "Army Intelligence Office"; Moore to Ann E. Gates, Nov. 22, 1864, 741(2)-VI-RG109; "Dudley Dunn Saunders."

24. Moore to Randolph, Sept. 5, 1862, enclosure in Moore to Seddon, Dec. 29, 1863, entry UD 176A, RG 109; *JCCSA*, Sept. 15, 1862, 5:380–81.

25. Marshall, "Letter from Dr. Marshall—The Homeless Invalids," *Richmond Whig and Public Advertiser*, Oct. 2, 1863; *JCCSA*, Dec. 28, 1863, 6:568; Moore to Seddon, Dec. 29, 1863, entry UD 176A, RG 109; Marshall "Help for the Wounded—An Important Proposition," *Daily Richmond Enquirer*, Jan. 14, 1864; *JCCSA*, Feb. 13, 1864, 6:808–9.

26. Hasegawa, *Mending Broken Soldiers*, 46–69.

27. Hasegawa, *Mending Broken Soldiers*, 50–51; SO 279(15), Nov. 24, 1863, 15-I-RG109.

28. Payne, "Samuel Preston Moore's Letters."

29. Holloway, "Reminiscences."

30. Moore to Miles, Dec. 14, 1861, Mar. 24, 1862, entry UD 176A, RG 109; Moore, "Confederate Doctors," *Daily Dispatch* (Richmond), Oct. 20, 1875.

31. Estill, "Diary of a Confederate Congressman," 274n7, 294; Roberts to Cooper, Apr. 12, 1863, file for Roberts, microfilm M331(213); Moore to Speaker

of the House, Jan. 10, 1863, entry UD 176A, RG 109; Georgian [pseud.], letter, *Daily Richmond Examiner,* Sept. 23, 1862; Jones, *Rebel War Clerk's Diary,* 1:210.

32. "Medical Department," *Daily Enquirer* (Richmond), Apr. 11, 1863.
33. Rowland, *Jefferson Davis, Constitutionalist,* 376.

3. Medical Directors

1. Bartholomees, *Buff Facings and Gilt Buttons,* 71; Epstein, "Creation and Evolution of the Army Corps," 21–26; War Department (Confederate), *Army Regulations* (1861), 56.
2. War Department (Confederate), *Regulations for the Medical Department* (1861), 3.
3. GO 1–8, Army of the Mississippi, Mar. 29, 1862, *OR,* ser. 1, 10(2):370–71; Lawrence to Hardee, Apr. 11, 13, 14, 1862, Lawrence to Thomas Jordan, Apr. 18, 1862, and Hardee to Cooper, May 8, 1862, all with endorsements, file for Lawrence, microfilm M331(153).
4. GO 1–8, Army of the Mississippi, Mar. 29, 1862, *OR,* ser. 1, 10(2):370–71; Lawrence to Hardee, Apr. 11, 13, 14, 1862, Lawrence to Thomas Jordan, Apr. 18, 1862, and Hardee to Cooper, May 8, 1862, all with endorsements, file for Lawrence, microfilm M331(153); War Department (Confederate), *Regulations for the Medical Department* (Apr. 10, 1862); George W. Randolph, orders, Mar. 26, 1862, *OR,* ser. 4, 1:1024–25.
5. Surgeon General's Office, circular, Aug. 18, 1862, *OR,* ser. 4, 2:56; GO 78, Oct. 28, 1862, 2-I-RG109.
6. Moore to Foard, May 7, 1862, file for Moore, microfilm M331(181); Moore to Edwin S. Gaillard, Nov. 6, 1862, 739(2)-VI-RG109.
7. Moore to Gaillard, Oct. 10, 1862, 739(2)-VI-RG109; GO 124(3), Sept. 22, 1863, 3-I-RG109.
8. Stout, "Some Facts" (Nov. 1902), 624; Hines to Gaillard, Sep. 30, 1862, file for Hines, microfilm M331(128).
9. Roberts, "Organization and Personnel"; GO 23(1), Feb. 25, 1863, 3-I-RG109; War Department (Confederate), *Regulations for the Medical Department* (Mar. 25, 1863), 5; Holloway to Moore, Apr. 4, 1863, file C843, microfilm M437(87).
10. Hardee to Mackall, June 20, 1863, file for Johnson, microfilm M331(131).
11. Heustis to Breckinridge, Oct. 28, 1863, file for Heustis, microfilm M331 (125).
12. GO 28(5), Mar. 12, 1863, 3-I-RG109.

13. Samuel Cooper to James A. Seddon, Nov. 15, 1864, *OR*, ser. 4, 3:836–37; GO 44, Apr. 29, 1864, 203-I-RG109; Surgeon General's Office, circular, Aug. 18, 1862, *OR*, ser. 4, 2:56; Act of June 14, 1864, chap. 58, Cong. C.S.A. Stat. 281.

14. Roberts, "Organization and Personnel."

15. Williams to Moore, Nov. 23, 1861, 367-VI-RG109; Guild to Moore, Aug. 16, 1862, *OR*, ser. 1, 11(2):501–2.

16. Moore to Foard, May 7, 1862, file for Moore, microfilm M331(181); Carrington to Fitzgerald, Dec. 21, 1864, 364-VI-RG109.

17. "Army Medical Intelligence" (Sept. 1864).

18. GO 28(5), Mar. 12, 1863, 3-I-RG109; Moore to Cooper, July 17, 1863, with endorsements, file S1465, microfilm M474(82); SO 65, Mar. 17, 1863, 207-I-RG109; GO 23(1), Feb. 25, 1863, 3-I-RG109; War Department (Confederate), *Regulations for the Medical Department* (Mar. 25, 1863), 5.

19. Moore to Seddon, Mar. 7, Apr. 7, 1863, file C843, microfilm M437(87); Moore to AIGO, Mar. 21, 1863, letter S635, 54-I-RG109; SO 80(1, 2), Apr. 2, 1863, 207-I-RG109.

20. Cooper, statement, Apr. 14, 1863, file C843, microfilm M437(87). As medical director of hospitals, Carrington first occupied space at 213 Main Street, near Ninth Street and only half a block from the Mechanics Institute building, which housed the SGO. By April 21, 1863, he moved to Ninth Street, just two doors north of the Mechanics Institute. By late September 1863 Carrington moved to the so-called Winder Building, a new structure on the southwest corner of Tenth Street and Broad Streets. Although never far from the SGO, he was not considered part of the SGO staff. Carrington to surgeon in charge, Smallpox Hospital, Apr. 21, 1863, file for Carrington, microfilm M331(49); *Stranger's Guide*, 3, 10–11; Circular, Sept. 28, 1863, 7-VI-RG109.

21. SO 80(1), Apr. 2, 1863, 207-I-RG109; Vance to Seddon, Sept. 3, 1863, *OR*, ser. 4, 2:787–88.

22. Carrington to surgeon in charge, Howard's Grove Hospital, Mar. 19, 1863, file for Carrington, microfilm M331(49); Carrington to Moore, Apr. 14, 1863, 416-VI-RG109.

23. Moore to Cooper, Sept. 4, 1863, file S1794, microfilm M474(83); SO 211(7), Sept. 5, 1863, 14-I-RG109.

24. SO 276(5), Nov. 20, 1863, 208-I-RG109; Ross to Cooper (two letters), Nov. 28, 1863, and Maury to Cooper, Nov. 29, 1863, with endorsements, file for Ross, microfilm M331(216).

25. Smith to James H. Berrien, Aug. 22, 1863, file for Smith, microfilm M331 (231).

26. Heustis to Cooper, Apr. 28, 1863, with endorsements, file for Heustis, microfilm M331(125); "Army Medical Intelligence" (Sept. 1864).

27. Headquarters, Dept. No. 2, SO 160(6), Aug. 22, 1863, file for Stout, microfilm M331(237); Schroeder-Lein, *Confederate Hospitals on the Move*, 64–68; SO 99(24), Apr. 23, 1863, SO 115(11), May 14, 1863, and SO 128(2, 3), May 29, 1863, 207-I-RG109; Stout, "Some Facts" (May 1903), 276–77.

28. Stout, "Some Facts" (May 1903), 279; Moore to Foard, May 13, 1863, 748-VI-RG109.

29. Polk to Cooper, Apr. 10, 1863, *OR*, ser. 1, 23(2):747–49; Stout, "Some Facts" (May 1903), 278.

30. Guild to Walter H. Taylor, Jan. 5, 1863, 641-VI-RG109; Cavalry Division, Army of Northern Virginia, SO 51(1), Feb. 21, 1863, file for Eliason, microfilm M331(85).

31. Moore to Cooper, Nov. 6, 1863, file S2334, microfilm M474(84).

32. Moore to Cooper, July 17, 1863, with endorsements, file S1465, microfilm M474(82).

33. "Army Medical Intelligence" (Sept. 1864); SO 70, Mar. 21, 1863, SO 80(1, 2), Apr. 2, 1863, SO 88(1), Apr. 10, 1863, and SO 128(3), May 29, 1863, 207-I-RG109; SO 27(5), Feb. 2, 1864, 16-I-RG109; SO 155(5), July 4, 1864, 18-I-RG109.

4. Medical Inspectors

1. Moore to William Porcher Miles, Mar. 24, 1862, entry UD 176A, RG 109.

2. War Department (Confederate), *Regulations for the Medical Department* (1861), 3; War Department (Confederate), *Army Regulations*, 29, 32, 56; T. N. Waul, Report, Jan. 29, 1862, *JCCSA*, 1:720–27.

3. SO 117(4), Aug. 7, 1861, 6-I-RG109.

4. Moore to Elisha P. Langworthy, Sept. 12, 1861, file for Langworthy, microfilm M331(152); Moore to Thomas H. Williams, Sept. 12, 1861, 739 (1)-VI-RG109.

5. T. N. Waul, Report, Jan. 29, 1862, *JCCSA*, 1:720–27; Moore to William Porcher Miles, Mar. 24, 1862, entry UD 176A, RG 109.

6. Gaillard to George W. Randolph, Sept. 3, 1862, entry UD 176A, RG 109.

7. T. N. Waul, Report, Jan. 29, 1862, *JCCSA*, 1:720–27; Peachy to Gaillard, Sept. 29, 1862, file for Peachy, microfilm M331(195).

8. SO 261(17), Dec. 9, 1861, and SO 266(15), Dec. 14, 1861, 204-I-RG109; SO 125(13), May 31, 1862, and SO 130(5, 6), June 6, 1862, 9-I-RG109; SO

104(3, 4), Apr. 29, 1863, and SO 107(12), May 2, 1863, 13-I-RG109; SO 167(4), July 13, 1863, and SO 170(4), July 18, 1863, 218-I-RG109; SO 70(7), Mar. 21, 1863, 12-I-RG109; SO 246(2), Oct. 16, 1863, 15-I-RG109.

9. GO 119(3), Sept. 7, 1863, 3-I-RG109; SO 226(3, 4), Sept. 23, 1863, and SO 228(3), Sept. 25, 1863, 218-I-RG109; Moore to Edward A. Flewellen, Sept. 11, 1863, 748-VI-RG109; Moore to William A. Carrington, Jan. 14, 1864, 741(1)-VI-RG109.

10. Samuel Cooper to James A. Seddon, Nov. 15, 1864, *OR*, ser. 4, 3:836; GO 44, Apr. 29, 1864, 203-I-RG109.

11. "Army Medical Intelligence" (Sept. 1864); SO 167(4), July 13, 1863, and SO 170, July 18, 1863, 218-I-RG109; SO 246(2), Oct. 16, 1863, and SO 260(6), Nov. 2, 1863, 15-I-RG109; SO 242(18), Oct. 16, 1862, 11-I-RG109; SO 44(15), Feb. 23, 1864, 16-I-RG109; SO 218(18), Sept. 14, 1864, 18-I-RG109.

12. Saunders, inspection report, Dec. 1864–Jan. 1865, report S-45, microfilm M935(17); Carrington to Samuel Cooper, Feb. 11, 1865, file for Carrington, microfilm M331(49); Robert H. Chilton to Carrington, Feb. 23, 1865, file for Chilton, microfilm M331(54).

13. Moore to Clopton, Jan. 21, 1865, entry UD 176A, RG 109.

14. SO 107(12), May 2, 1863, 13-I-RG109; *Stranger's Guide*, 11; Return of Civil and Military Officers, file 3055, entry 183, RG 109.

5. Medical Purveyors

1. SO 32(6), Apr. 22, 1861, SO 44(7), May 6, 1861, and SO 92(4), July 9, 1861, 6-I-RG109; Department of Texas, GO 2, May 1, 1861, file for Howard, microfilm M331(133); Department of Texas, GO 11, June 17, 1861, file for Langworthy, microfilm M331(152); SO 196(7), Oct. 30, 1861, 204-I-RG109; War Department (Confederate), *Regulations for the Medical Department* (1861), 4.

2. SO 196(7), Oct. 30, 1861, 204-I-RG109; Chisolm, orders, Nov. 8, 19, 1861, Chisolm to W. H. Cumming, Dec. 12, 1861, and Chisolm to Moore, Feb. 28, 1862, "Letter Book of Medical Director's Office, " Wessels Library; SO 55(13), Mar. 10, 1862, 8-I-RG109; War Department (Confederate), *Regulations for the Medical Department* (Apr. 10, 1862).

3. SO 64(2), June 5, 1861, 6-I-RG109; War Department (Confederate), *Regulations for the Medical Department* (1861), 4; War Department (Confederate), *Regulations for the Army* (Mar. 13, 1862), 236; War Department (Confederate), *Regulations for the Army* (Jan. 28, 1863), 234; Roberts, "Confederate Medical Service," 349; Moore to John Withers, Apr. 7, 1862, file S639, microfilm M474(46); SO 79(6), Apr. 7, 1861, and SO 80(2), Apr. 8, 1861, 9-I-RG109.

4. Johns, Circular No. 1, Apr. 12, 1862, Circular No. 3, Apr. 25, 1862, Circular No. 6, June 11, 1862, and Johns to Edwin S. Gaillard, Oct. 18, 1862, file for Johns, microfilm M346(506).

5. *Stranger's Guide*, 10; Williams, "Reminiscences," 301; Unsigned document with endorsement by Jefferson Davis, Mar. 7, 1863, *OR*, ser. 4, 2:421–24; Chisolm to Johns, May 30, 1862, "Letter Book of Dr. J. J. Chisolm," Wessels Library.

6. Prioleau to Johns, Aug. 14, 1862, Prioleau to Moore, Sept. 8, 1862, and Prioleau to George S. Blackie, Sept. 15, 1862, 572-VI-RG109; Moore to Prioleau, Aug. 21, 1862, Johns to Prioleau, Sept. 5, 1862, and Moore to Prioleau, Oct. 2, 1862, 566-VI-RG109; Johns, Circular No. 17, Sept. 11, 1862, 135-VI-RG109.

7. Unsigned document with endorsement by Davis, Mar. 7, 1863, *OR*, ser. 4, 2:421–24; Moore to AIGO, Jan. 28, 1863, letter S-189, 54-I-RG109.

8. "Medical Department of the Confederate States Army."

9. Return of Civil and Military Officers, file 3055, entry 183, RG 109; Roberts, "Confederate Medical Service," 241; SO 11(24), Jan. 14, 1863, 207-I-RG109.

10. "Confederate Congress," *Daily Richmond Examiner*, Mar. 13, 1863; "Medical Purveyors—the Rank of Surgeons," *Daily Richmond Examiner*, Apr. 13, 1863.

11. Johns, Circular No. 3, Apr. 12, 1862, file for Johns, microfilm M346(506); Johns, Circular No. 13, Aug. 22, 1862, 135-VI-RG109; Consolidated Report of Persons Employed . . . , Nov. 10, 1864, file S-3285, microfilm M474(145); Consolidated Report of Persons Employed . . . , Feb. 1865, file C-277, microfilm M474(155); Miller to Second Auditor, Richmond, July 13, 1863, file for F. C. Goodgame, 18th Alabama Infantry, microfilm M311(265).

12. SO 92(4), July 9, 1861, 204-I-RG109; Potts, "Medical Department, C.S. Army," *Daily Appeal* (Memphis), Mar. 30, 1862; Johns, Circular No. 3, Apr. 12, 1862, file for Johns, microfilm M346(506); Scott to Thomas M. Jack, Jan. 7, 1864, file for Potts, microfilm M331(201).

13. Potts to Moore, July 30, 1864, with endorsements, file for Potts, microfilm M331(201).

14. Potts to Moore, July 30, 1864, with endorsements.

15. Moore to Seddon, July 25, 1864, with endorsements, file S2073, microfilm M474(143).

16. Moore to Cooper, Aug. 17, 1864, file S2185, microfilm M474(143); SO 197(4), Aug. 20, 1864, 18-I-RG109.

17. Johns to William H. Prioleau, Apr. 30, 1862, 6-VI-RG109; Johns to J. J. Chisolm, May 3, 1862, file for Johns, microfilm M346(506); Moore to Prioleau,

July 15, 1864, and Moore to George Blackie, July 28, 1864, 628-VI-RG109; "Exciting News from Jackson," *Daily Chronicle & Sentinel* (Augusta, GA), May 19, 1863; Moore to Potts, June 3, 1863, 740(1)-VI-RG109; Prioleau, advertisement, *Macon (GA) Daily Telegraph & Confederate*, Feb. 25, 1865; Blackie, advertisements, July 1, Aug. 4, 1864, *Daily Constitutionalist* (Augusta, GA).

18. Johns, Circular No. 3, Apr. 12, 1862, file for Johns, microfilm M346(506); W. H. Geddings to Herndon, Oct. 8, 1862, file for Herndon, microfilm M331(125).

19. Consolidated Report of Persons Employed . . . , Nov. 10, 1864, file S-3285, microfilm M474(145); Consolidated Report of Persons Employed . . . , Feb. 1865, file C-277, microfilm M474(155); "Army Medical Intelligence" (Nov. 1864).

20. Hasegawa and Hambrecht, "Confederate Medical Laboratories."

21. Johns to Moore, Jan. 22, 1862, file S246, microfilm M474(45); SO 36(2), Feb. 3, 1862, 205-I-RG109; Sengstack to unknown, July 23, 1863, file for Sengstack, microfilm M324(360); SO 288(3), Dec. 9, 1862, 206-I-RG109; Moore to Richard Potts, June 6, 1863, 740(1)-VI-RG109; Hasegawa and Hambrecht, "Confederate Medical Laboratories."

22. Hasegawa and Hambrecht, "Confederate Medical Laboratories"; Moore, Consolidated Report of Persons Employed . . . , Nov. 14, 1864, file S3285, microfilm M427(145); Williams, "Reminiscences"; Hasegawa, "Absurd Prejudice."

23. SO 274(20–22, 24–26), Nov. 18, 1864, 210-I-RG109; Robert Tyler to James A. Seddon, June 1, 1864, file T128, microfilm M437(143); Lee to Samuel Cooper, Nov. 29, 1864, entry L1582, 68-I-RG109.

24. Moore to Breckinridge, Feb. 9, 1865, *OR*, ser. 4. 3:1073–76.

25. Moore to Breckinridge, Feb. 9, 1865; Moore to William H. Prioleau, Feb. 23, 1863, 740(1)-VI-RG109; "Army Medical Intelligence" (Oct. 1864); Moore, "Confederate Doctors," *Daily Dispatch* (Richmond), Oct. 20, 1875.

6. Importation of Medical Supplies

1. Davis, *Rise and Fall of the Confederate Government*, 1:310; Moore, "Confederate Doctors," *Daily Dispatch* (Richmond), Oct. 20, 1875; War Department (US), *Regulations for the Medical Department of the Army*, 17–32; War Department (Confederate), *Army Regulations* (1861), 194–96; War Department (US), *Regulations for the Army of the United States*, 249–50; Act of Mar. 6, 1861, chap. 29, § 29, Prov. Cong. C.S.A. Stat. 47, 51; War Department (Confederate), *Regulations for the Medical Department of the*

Confederate States Army, 13–22; War Department (Confederate), *Regulations for the Medical Department of the C.S. Army* (1862 and 1863), 16–27.

2. T. O. Edwards to R. C. Winthrop, Dec. 26, 1848, H. Exec. Doc. 43, 30th Cong., 2nd sess., 1849, 2; Squibb, "Drug Inspectors"; Freedley, *Leading Pursuits,* 113–35; Zeilin, "Drug Business."

3. England, "American Manufacture of Quinine Sulphate"; Cole, "Manufacture and Consumption of Quinine."

4. "Commercial Dependence of the South on the North"; Wise, *Lifeline of the Confederacy,* 12; *Report of the Secretary of the Treasury,* 474–75; Wood and Co., "Review of the Drug Trade"; Wood and Nichols, "Annual Report on Drugs"; Wood and Nichols, "Annual Report on the Drug Trade"; Act of Feb. 18, 1861, chap. 3, § 2, Prov. Cong. C.S.A. Stat. 28; Act of Feb. 26, 1861, chap. 16, Prov. Cong. C.S.A. Stat. 38; Zeilin, "Drug Business."

5. Nichols, "Review of the New York Markets"; Basler, *Collected Works of Abraham Lincoln,* 338–39, 346–47, 487–88; "What Articles Are Contraband of War," *Boston Evening Transcript,* May 16, 1861; "No Drugs South!," *Boston Evening Transcript,* June 1, 1861; Leigh, *Trading with the Enemy,* 15.

6. Edmonson, *American Surgical Instruments,* 43–130, 170–269.

7. Wise, *Lifeline of the Confederacy;* Thompson, *Confederate Purchasing Operations Abroad.*

8. Huse, *Supplies for the Confederate Army,* 9–10; Samuel Cooper to Huse, Apr. 15, 1861, *OR,* ser. 4, 1:220; Gorgas to James A. Seddon, May 22, 1863, ibid., 2:564.

9. Moore to Blackie, June 27, July 13, 1862, and Moore to Seixas, July 9, 1862, 750-VI-RG109; Moore to Huse, June 29, 1863, file for Huse, microfilm M331(137); Moore to Huse, Aug. 22, Oct. 14, 1863, *Correspondence Concerning Claims,* 64, 71.

10. Walker to Gifford and Tucker, July 26, 1861, microfilm M522(1); Gifford and Tucker to Walker, Aug. 1, 1861, file 2998, microfilm M437(6); Myers to Benjamin, Oct. 1, 1861, Gifford and Tucker to Myers, Oct. 1, 1861, and Tucker, memorandum, n.d., file 6317, microfilm M437(11); Tucker to George W. Randolph, Sept. 19, 1862, *OR,* ser. 4, 2:87–89. There have been various rendering of Gifford's given name, including Adolphus (or Augustus) Frederick Daubeny; the initials often appear incorrectly as "A. T. D." in published sources. Tucker rarely used his first name of Nathaniel.

11. Tucker to Randolph, Sept. 9, 1862, *OR,* ser. 4, 2:87–89; "Departure of the Bermuda," *Savannah Republican,* Nov. 4, 1861; Tucker, *Beverly Tucker,* 18; Tucker to James A. Seddon, July 15, 1863, file T147, microfilm M347(398); Ludwell H. Johnson, "Beverly Tucker's Canadian Mission."

12. Death notice for Evans, *Wilmington (NC) Journal,* Mar. 12, 1863; *Catalogue of Alumni,* 55; Evans to Walker, July 2, 1861, microfilm M437(4); Evans to Walker, July 10, 1861, microfilm M437(6); Evans to Randolph, Oct. 4, 1862, file E176, microfilm M437(45); Benjamin to Huse, Mar. 22, 1862, *OR,* ser. 4, 1:1018.

13. Evans to Eliza Evans, Oct. 29, 1861, and Jan. 1, 1862, Augustus Coutanche Evans Papers, Wilson Library; Evans to Randolph, Oct. 4, 1862, file E176, microfilm M437(45); Moore to Benjamin, Mar. 6, 1862, file M222, microfilm M437(59); Benjamin to Huse, Mar. 22, 1862, *OR,* ser. 4, 1:1018; Death notice for Evans, *Wilmington (NC) Journal,* Mar. 12, 1863.

14. Vandiver, *Confederate Blockade Running,* xxi–xxii, xxxii, 78–79, 88.

15. Adams, *Great Britain and the American Civil War,* 268–69n1; Barney to Salmon P. Chase, Aug. 9, 1862, H. Exec. Doc. 1, 37th Cong., 3rd sess., 1862, 276–77; Testimony of Epes Sargent, H. Rep. 111, 38th Cong., 1st sess., 1864, 273–74; Soley, *Blockade and the Cruisers,* 41–42; Wise, *Lifeline of the Confederacy,* 132, 191, 195.

16. Chisolm to Moore, Nov. 30, Dec. 7, 1861, "Letter Book of Medical Director's Office," Wessels Library; Wise, *Lifeline of the Confederacy,* 62; Chisolm to Johns, Sept. 1, 1862, Chisolm to Louis C. Heyliger, Sept. 12, 1862, Chisolm to R. T. Walker, Sept. 13, 1862, and Chisolm to John Lafitte, Sept. 13, 1862, "Letter Book of Dr. J. J. Chisolm," Wessels Library; Johns, Circular No. 1, Apr. 12, 1862, and Circular No. 3, Apr. 25, 1862, file for Johns, microfilm M346(506).

17. Moore to Prioleau, July 11, 1862, and Johns to Prioleau, July 13 (telegram), July 28, Aug. 4 1862, 566-VI-RG109; Prioleau to Johns, July [8, 9, or 10?], 1862, and Prioleau to Moore, July 17, 1862, 572-VI-RG109.

18. Talley to Moore, Oct. 8, 1861, "Letter Book of Medical Director's Office," Wessels Library; Prioleau to Johns, June 28, July 10, 1862, 572-VI-RG109.

19. Johns to Prioleau, July 5, 1862, 566-VI-RG109.

20. Johns to Prioleau, July 4, 1862, with copy of Randolph endorsement, June 19, 1862, 566-VI-RG109.

21. Ashhurst to Prioleau, July 2, 8, 12, 1862, 566-VI-RG109; Prioleau to Johns, July 14, 1862, 572-VI-RG109.

22. Chisolm to Edmondston, May 27, 1862, "Letter Book of Dr. J. J. Chisolm," Wessels Library.

23. Chisolm to Edmondston, May 27, 1862, Chisolm to Johns, May 31, 1862, Chisolm to Prioleau, May 31, 1862, and Chisolm to Johns, Sept. 13, 1862, "Letter Book of Dr. J. J. Chisolm," Wessels Library.

24. Wise, *Lifeline of the Confederacy,* 262; Moore to Blackie, Feb. 12, 19, 1863, Davidson to Blackie, Apr. 6, 1863, and William Flash to Blackie, May 27, 1862, 750-VI-RG109.

25. Prioleau to Johns, May 27, 1862, 572-VI-RG109; Chisolm to unknown, Nov. 10, 1862, "Letter Book of Dr. J. J. Chisolm," Wessels Library.

26. Johnson, "Trading with the Union"; C. C. Washburn, Department of West Tennessee, GO 3, May 10, 1864, *OR*, ser. 1, 39(2):22–23.

27. Covey to Moore, Oct. 4, 1863, James King Hall Papers, Wilson Library; Covey to Potts, Oct. 13, 1864, with extract of letter, Oct. 4, 1864, file for Covey, microfilm M331(63).

28. Potts to Moore, Aug. 30, 1864, and Potts to Miller, Sept. 26, 1864, 629-VI-RG109.

29. Moore to John C. Breckinridge, Feb. 9, 1865, *OR*, ser. 4, 3:1073–76; Potts to Moore, Feb. 16, 1865, 629-VI-RG109; Wise, *Lifeline of the Confederacy*, 241.

30. James A. Seddon to Lucius J. Gartrell, Mar. 3, 1863, microfilm M522(6).

31. Moore, SO, July 6, 1863, file S1409, microfilm M474(82); SO 161(18), July 8, 1863, 218-I-RG109.

32. John A. Campbell, permits, Oct. 16, 27, 1863, microfilm M522(8); John W. Oslin and Charles E. V. Nickerson to General Beauregard's Corps, May 17, 1864, with endorsements, file for Crawford, M331(65); SO 214(16), Sept. 9, 1864, 18-I-RG109; Balderston to Andrew Johnson, Aug. 26, 1865, file for Balderston, microfilm M1003(30), RG 94; Balderston to Seddon, Jan. 1, 1865, file B180, microfilm M474(153); CSR for Fedderman, microfilm M324(850).

33. File for Fedderman, microfilm M345(90); "Sentence of a Blockade Runner," *Evening Star* (Washington, DC), July 25, 1864; John A. Fisher to E. D. Townsend, June 27, 1864, file F225, microfilm M619(256), RG 94; Henry A. Lockwood to Lincoln, Mar. 2, 1865, with endorsements, file F173, M619(353), RG 94.

7. Turning to Domestic Resources

1. Act of Aug. 2, 1861, chap. 7, Prov. Cong. C.S.A. Stat. 170; Johns, notice, *Richmond Enquirer*, June 10, 1862.

2. Chisolm to Prioleau, Mar. 29, 1862, 6-VI-RG109; Prioleau to Johns, Apr. 22, 1862, 572-VI-RG109.

3. Prioleau to Johns, Apr. 23, 1862, 572-VI-RG109; Johns to Prioleau, Apr. 30, 1862, 6-VI-RG109.

4. Johns, Circular No. 3, Apr. 25, 1862, file for Johns, microfilm M346(506).

5. Chisolm to Blackie, Feb. 2, 1863, 750-VI-RG109; Stewart to Prioleau, Aug. 13, 1862, file for Stewart, microfilm M346(983); Blackie to Prioleau, Aug. 23, 1862, file for Blackie, microfilm M331(24); Chisolm to Prioleau, May 31, 1862, "Letter Book of Dr. J. J. Chisolm," Wessels Library.

6. Alexander N. Talley, "To Members of the Medical Profession," *Charleston (SC) Mercury*, Oct. 1, 1861; Edward Warren, notice, *Fayetteville (NC) Observer*, July 7, 1862; Prioleau to Johns, Apr. 23, 1862, 572-VI-RG109; Johns to Prioleau, Apr. 30, 1862, 6-VI-RG109; Johns to Prioleau, Aug. 13, 1862, 566-VI-RG109.

7. Chisolm to Charles Edmondston, June 2, 1862, "Letter Book of Dr. J. J. Chisolm," Wessels Library; R. A. Kinloch to Benjamin & Goodrich, Nov. 14, 1861, and Chisolm to H. B. Horlbeck, June 23, 1862, "Letter Book of Medical Director's Office," ibid.; McKensie, receipt, June 25, 1861, file for McKensie, microfilm M346(634); Benjamin & Goodrich, invoice, Nov. 27, 1861, file for Benjamin & Goodrich, microfilm M346(58); Thauss, invoice, Mar. 12, 1863, file for Thauss, microfilm M346(1018); Accounts for Straus and Oliver & Douglass, 623-VI-RG109; "Home Manufactures and Industry," *Southerner* (Tarboro, NC), May 23, 1863; Holtzscheiter, advertisement, *Southerner* (Tarboro, NC), Sept. 1, 1860; "A Handsome Sword," *Daily Confederate* (Raleigh, NC), Apr. 13, 1864; Johns to Samuel Cooper, May 26, 1864, file L665, microfilm M474(125); "March of Improvement," *Sentinel* (Richmond), Mar. 30, 1864; Guild to Moore, Apr. 14, 1863, 641-VI-RG109; Moore, "Confederate Doctors," *Daily Dispatch* (Richmond), Oct. 20, 1875.

8. Johns to AIGO, Apr. 1, 1862, file M692, microfilm M474(33); Accounts for Gustin, Wood, and Marshall, 623-VI-RG109.

9. Moore to John C. Breckinridge, Feb. 9, 1865, *OR*, ser. 4, 3:1073–76; Moore, Consolidated Report of Persons Employed . . . , Nov. 15, 1864, file S3285, microfilm M474(145); Moore to Prioleau, July 9, 1864, 628-VI-RG109.

10. Joseph C. G. Kennedy, *Preliminary Report on the Eighth Census, 1860*, S. Rep. (unnumbered), 37th Cong., 2nd sess., 1862, 178; Chisolm to Johns, June 7, 1862, "Letter Book of Dr. J. J. Chisolm," Wessels Library; Moore to Breckinridge, Feb. 9, 1865, *OR*, ser. 4, 3:1073–76.

11. Moore to Prioleau, Mar. 18, 1863, 740(1)-VI-RG109; J. F. Cummings to Lucius B. Northrop, Feb. 13, 1864, with enclosures, *OR*, ser. 4, 3:115–20; Vance to James A. Seddon, Dec. 31, 1863, with endorsements, ibid., 2:1072–73; Act of June 14, 1864, chap. 41, Cong. C.S.A. Stat. 271; Moore to Breckinridge, Feb. 9, 1865, *OR*, ser. 4, 3:1073–76; Moore, Consolidated Report of Persons Employed . . . , Nov. 14, 1864, file S3285, microfilm M427(145); Moore, Consolidated Report of Persons Employed . . . , Feb. 1865, file C277, microfilm M474(155); John B. Bond to John M. Haden, June 15, 1864, file for Bond, microfilm M331(27); William R. Johnston, Report of Operations CS Chemical Laboratory, Tyler, TX, file for Johnston, microfilm M331(142).

12. Moore, "Confederate Doctors," *Daily Dispatch* (Richmond), Oct. 20, 1875; Hasegawa, "Southern Resources"; Moore to Prioleau, Sept. 16, 1863, 566-VI-RG109; George W. Sites to George S. Barnsley, June 5, 1863, *George Scarborough Barnsley Papers*. In the context of Confederate medicinal flora, "indigenous" plants were native or introduced and could be growing in the wild or cultivated.

13. Chisolm to S. and E. Levy, Dec. 14, 1861, and Chisolm to Johns, Dec. 28, 1861, "Letter Book of Dr. J. J. Chisolm," Wessels Library; Prioleau to Johns, Apr. 23. 1862, 572-VI-RG109.

14. *General Directions*; Moore, circular, Apr. 2, 1862, *OR*, ser. 4, 1:1041; Johns, Circular No. 3, Apr. 25, 1862, file for Johns, microfilm M346(506).

15. Moore, circulars, Sept. 9, 17, 20, 1862, and Johns, circular, Aug. 11, 1862, 135-VI-RG109; Moore to Prioleau, Sept. 16, 1862, 566-VI-RG109; Prioleau to Johns, Aug. 18, 1862, 572-VI-RG109; Moore to Prioleau, June 9, 1863, 740(1)-VI-RG109.

16. Moore, circular, Apr. 23, 1863, 135-VI-RG109; Johnson, notice, *Western Democrat* (Charlotte, NC), Dec. 29, 1863; Chisolm, notice, *Charleston (SC) Mercury*, July 11, 1863; LeConte to unknown, Sept. 28, 1863, Papers of Aaron Snowden Piggot, RG 109.

17. Moore to Potts, Sept. 13, 1862, 740(2)-VI-RG109 (misfiled).

18. Mayes to Chisolm, Apr. 16, 1864, with endorsement, 709-VI-RG109.

19. Hasegawa, "Southern Resources"; *Standard Supply Table of Indigenous Remedies*.

20. Moore to Prioleau, Sept. 16, 1862, 566-VI-RG109; Prioleau to Moore, Sept. 24, 1862, 572-VI-RG109; Park, notice, *Savannah Republican*, Oct. 3, 1862.

21. Moore to Prioleau, Jan. 31, Apr. 23, 1863, 740(1)-VI-RG109; Moore, circular, and Moore to Prioleau, Dec. 5, 1862, 739(2)-VI-RG109.

22. Moore, "Confederate Doctors," *Daily Dispatch* (Richmond), Oct. 20, 1875; Moore to Prioleau, Oct. 17, 1862, 566-VI-RG109; Moore to Prioleau, Apr. 23, 1863, 740(1)-VI-RG109; Prioleau to Moore, Apr. 27, 1863, 627-VI-RG109; Hasegawa, "Quinine Substitutes"; Maury, "Hypodermic Injections."

23. Moore, circular, Mar. 19, 1863, *OR*, ser. 4, 2:442; News item, *Charleston (SC) Mercury*, May 29, 1863; "Opium," *Daily Chronicle & Sentinel* (Augusta, GA), June 10, 1863; Medicus [pseud.], "The Cultivation of Medicinal Plants," *Daily Constitutionalist* (Augusta, GA), Mar. 31, 1865; "Poppy," *Tri-Weekly Telegraph* (Houston), Jan. 15, 1864; Moore, "Confederate Doctors," *Daily Dispatch* (Richmond), Oct. 20, 1875; "Discussion on Opium."

24. *General Directions*; Parrish and Bakes, "Notes on Lactucarium"; Howard Smith, notice, *Arkansas State Gazette* (Little Rock), Nov. 29, 1862; Marion Howard, notice, *Fayetteville (NC) Observer*, Aug. 4, 1862.

25. Moore to Breckinridge, Feb. 9, 1865, *OR*, ser. 4, 3:1073–76; Hasegawa and Hambrecht, "Confederate Medical Laboratories."

26. Chisolm, List of Ingredients . . . Quarter Ending 30th Sept. 1863, file for Chisolm, microfilm M331(54); Voucher, May 3, 1863, file for J. J. Cohen, microfilm M346(180); "Save the Rose Leaves," *Daily Constitutionalist* (Augusta, GA), Apr. 25, 1863; Hasegawa and Hambrecht, "Confederate Medical Laboratories."

27. Hasegawa, "'Absurd Prejudice'"; Hasegawa and Hambrecht, "Confederate Medical Laboratories."

28. Hasegawa, "'Absurd Prejudice'"; Hasegawa, "Southern Resources"; "Brief Paragraphs," *Alexandria (VA) Gazette*, Aug. 28, 1863.

8. Care on and near the Battlefield

1. Cunningham, *Field Medical Services*, 23–41; "Meeting of Citizens for Relief of the Soldiers Wounded in the Late Battle," *Daily Dispatch* (Richmond), July 23, 1861.

2. War Department (US), *Regulations for the Army*; War Department (Confederate), *Army Regulations*; War Department (Confederate), *Regulations for the Army* (1864); Smart, "Transportation of Wounded in War."

3. J.L.C., "Southern Medicines," *Macon (GA) Daily Telegraph*, May 10, 1861; Larrey, *Memoirs*; "Soldier-Surgeon"; "French Field Hospitals"; Longmore, *Treatise on the Transport of Sick and Wounded*, 25–59. The French ambulance system was even described in a popular encyclopedia. See *New American Cyclopedia*, 1:451–52.

4. Moore to Walker, Aug. 19, 1861, file 3321, microfilm M437(7); Walker to Moore, Aug. 21, 1861, microfilm M522(2).

5. *JCCSA*, 1:368, 390–91; Davis to Miles, Aug. 19, 1861, Crist and Dix, *Papers of Jefferson Davis*, 288; Walker to Davis, Aug. 21, 1861, microfilm M522(2).

6. Moore to Miles, Dec. 14, 1861, entry UD 176A, RG 109.

7. Surgeon General's Office, circular, May 7, 1862, National Library of Medicine, http://resource.nlm.nih.gov/101644580 (accessed May 19, 2019); Aquia District, circular, Apr. 19, 1862, file for William A. Carrington, microfilm M331(49); Army of the Mississippi, General Orders No. 3, Mar. 14, 1862, *OR*, ser. 1, 10(2):325–26; "Important Army Order," *Daily Picayune* (New Orleans), Apr. 20, 1862.

8. William Barksdale to Andrew G. Dickinson, July 24, 1862, *OR*, ser. 1, 11(2): 750–52, E. C. Edmonds to R. H. Chilton, Aug. 15, 1862, ibid., 823–25; Benjamin Huger to R. E. Lee, July 21, 1862, ibid., 787–91; Hill to Chilton, Feb. 28, 1863, ibid., 834–40; Anderson to A. P. Hill, July 25, 1862, ibid., 877–81.

9. "The Ambulance Committee," *Daily Richmond Examiner*, June 12, 1862; "The Citizen Ambulance Corps of Richmond," ibid., Mar. 9, 1864; "The Ambulance Committee," *Daily Dispatch* (Richmond), June 22, 1866; Guild to Moore, Aug. 16, 1862, *OR*, ser. 1, 11(2):501–2; Guild to Moore, Dec. 15, 1862, 641-VI-RG109; GO 61, Aug. 23, 1862, 2-I-RG109.

10. Guild to Moore, Nov. 22, 1862, 641-VI-RG109.

11. Gaillard to Randolph, Sept. 3, 1862, entry UD 176A, RG 109; G. W. Smith to Thomas G. Rhett, June 23, 1862, *OR*, ser. 1, 11(2):989–94.

12. Gaillard to Randolph, Sept. 3, 1862, entry UD 176A, RG 109.

13. Randolph to Miles, Sept. 4, 1862, entry UD 176A, RG 109; *JCCSA*, 5:288–89, 384, 454, 486–87, 493; ibid., 2:379, 380–81, 405–6, 415.

14. Jefferson Davis, *Message of the President Vetoing the Medical Bill*, Oct. 13, 1862, Hathi Trust (source, Duke University), https://hdl.handle.net/2027/dul1.ark:/13960/t3mw3842c (accessed Aug. 9, 2019).

15. *JCCSA*, 3:155, 278–79; "The Confederate Congress: The Medical Department," *Daily Richmond Examiner*, Mar. 13, 1863.

16. *JCCSA*, 6:323–25; "Confederate States Congress: Medical Department," *Daily Enquirer* (Richmond), Apr. 11, 1863.

17. *JCCSA*, 6:463; ibid., 3:379.

18. Moore, Circular No. 5, Mar. 15, 1864, file for Carrington, microfilm M331 (49); Schroeder-Lein, *Confederate Hospitals on the Move*, 132–33.

19. Carrington to Johns, Apr. 26, May 3, 1864, and Carrington to Moore, May 24, 1864, 364-VI-RG109.

20. War Department (Confederate), *Regulations for the Medical Department* (1861), 57; War Department (Confederate), *Regulations for the Medical Department* (1862), 55; War Department (Confederate), *Regulations for the Medical Department* (1863), 57; Chisolm, *Manual of Military Surgery*, 3rd ed., 99–106.

21. Richard C. Macmurdo to R. V. Gaines, Jan. 16, 1865, microfilm M331(161); Quartermaster's voucher for Richard W. Birchett, Oct. 1, 1863, microfilm M346(66).

22. Letterman, *Medical Recollections*.

9. General Hospitals

1. Cunningham, *Doctors in Gray*, 45; Carrington to Moore, Apr. 14, 1863, 416-VI-RG109; Chisolm, *Manual of Military Surgery*, 3rd ed., 64. Cunningham's remark about the derivation of "general hospitals" is the apparent basis of historians saying that they "served any man regardless of state or regimental affiliation" or "were open to soldiers from every state." Hilde,

Worth a Dozen Men, 17–18; Berlin, *Confederate Nurse*, 7. Those interpretations are problematic in that many general hospitals were intended for the treatment of patients from particular states.

2. Rosenberg, *Care of Strangers*, 4–5; Blanton, *Medicine in Virginia*, 211–15; Calcutt, *Richmond's Wartime Hospitals*, 22–23.

3. "Hospital of St. Francis de Sales," *Daily Dispatch* (Richmond), May 3, 1861; "Nurses for the Army," ibid., June 10, 1861; "Meeting of Alabamians," *Daily Richmond Examiner*, Aug. 30, 1861; Buck, "Founder of the First Confederate Hospital"; Cunningham, *Doctors in Gray*, 184–217; "Sick Soldiers," *Daily Dispatch* (Richmond), June 1, 1861; "Hospital at Masons' Hall," ibid., July 1, 1861. Juliet Opie Hopkins was often identified as "Mrs. A. F. Hopkins" or "Mrs. Judge Hopkins." She was married to Arthur Francis Hopkins, a former chief justice of the Alabama Supreme Court and US senator. Griffith, "Mrs. Juliet Opie Hopkins."

4. Stout, "Some Facts" (Mar. 1902): 160–61.

5. Barnwell et al., *Report of the South Carolina Hospital Aid Association*; Vandiver, *Rebel Brass*, 6.

6. Carrington to Edwin S. Gaillard, Nov. 19, 1862, file for Carrington, microfilm M331(49); "List of the Sick and Wounded," *Richmond Enquirer*, July 31, 1861; "City Items: Sick and Wounded," *Richmond Whig and Public Advertiser*, July 30, 1861; "The Wounded," *Daily Dispatch* (Richmond), July 23, 1861; Moore, "Confederate Doctors," ibid., Oct. 20, 1875.

7. Smith to Walker, July 24, 1861, Magruder to Lee, July 18, 1861, and Walker to Miles, Aug. 7, 1861, entry UD 176A, RG 109; Moore to Walker, Aug. 9, 1861, file 2968, microfilm M437(6); Miles to Walker, Aug. 15, 1861, file 3175, microfilm M437(7); *JCCSA*, 1:364, 373, 384; Act of Aug. 21, 1861, chap. 29, Prov. Cong. C.S.A. Stat. 186.

8. Walker to Davis, Aug, 7, 1861, microfilm M522(2); Cunningham, *Field Medical Services*, 23–41, 69–91; Miles to Walker, Aug. 9, 1861, file 3042, microfilm M437(6); *JCCSA*, 1:374, 384; Act of Aug, 21, 1861, chap. 27, Prov. Cong. C.S.A. Stat. 186; Act of Aug. 21, 1861, chap. 32, Prov. Cong. C.S.A. Stat. 187.

9. Moore to Walker, Aug. 8, 1861, file 3174, microfilm M437(7); Benjamin to Moore, Oct. 16, 1861, microfilm M522(3).

10. *JCCSA*, 1:461–62.

11. "Report," *Daily Constitutionalist* (Augusta, GA), Dec. 8, 1861.

12. "Report," *Daily Constitutionalist* (Augusta, GA), Dec. 8, 1861; Georgia Relief and Hospital Association, *Report of the Executive Committee*, 29–30.

13. Carrington to Gaillard, Nov. 15, 1862, file for Carrington, microfilm M331(49); "Meeting of Alabamians," *Daily Richmond Examiner*, Aug. 30,

1861, 3; Calcutt, *Richmond's Wartime Hospitals*, 45–46, 134–35, 143–46; Barnwell et al., *Report of the South Carolina Hospital Aid Association*, 15–16; Williams to R. W. Barnwell, Nov. 12, 1861, 367-VI-RG109.

14. Norris, "For the Benefit of Our Gallant Volunteers"; *General Military Hospital for the North Carolina Troops*; SO 88(14), Apr. 17, 1862, 213-I-RG109; Index card, n.d., and Manson to James A. Seddon, Oct. 22, 1863, file for Manson, microfilm M331(163); Warren, "Report of the Surgeon General," *Daily Progress* (Raleigh), Dec. 1, 2, 1864. Wood was among those claiming a much more active role for North Carolina in establishing Moore Hospital. See Wood, "Otis Frederick Manson."

15. *JCCSA*, 1: 720–27; "The Hospital System in Richmond," *Daily Richmond Examiner*, Sept. 13, 1861, 2–3.

16. Moore, "Confederate Doctors," *Daily Dispatch* (Richmond), Oct. 20, 1875; Rosenberg, *Care of Strangers*, 122–41; *Addresses*, 16–19; Nightingale, *Notes on Hospitals*. Moore specified in 1863 that general hospitals should provide at least 800 cubic feet of space per bed, whereas Joseph Jones believed that a seriously wounded man needed at least 2,000 cubic feet. Moore, circular, July 6, 1863, Boston Athenaeum, http://catalog.bostonathenaeum.org/vwebv /holdingsInfo?bibId=325822 (accessed Sept. 8, 2018); Jones, "Investigations upon the Nature," 551. In anticipation of a large influx of sick and wounded soldiers into Richmond, Surgeon McCaw of Chimborazo Hospital was ordered to squeeze patients into his wards up to one per 500 cubic feet, if necessary. Carrington to McCaw, June 4, 1864, 709-VI-RG109.

17. "Chimborazo Hospital," *Richmond Whig and Public Advertiser*, Nov. 1, 1861; "The Hospital Service in Richmond—The 'Chimborazo Hospitals,'" *Daily Richmond Examiner*, Feb. 8, 1862; Moore, "Confederate Doctors," *Daily Dispatch* (Richmond), Oct. 20, 1875; Van Buren and Agnew, "Report No. 23"; Tripler to S. Williams, Sept. 9, 1861, *OR*, ser. 1, 5:100–101.

18. Newton, "My Recollections," 484; SO 129(30), June 5, 1862, 205-I-RG109; SO 54(2), Mar. 8, 1862, 213-I-RG109; Stout, "Some Facts" (Nov. 1902): 624, (Mar. 1903): 156, (May 1903): 276.

19. Moore, "Confederate Doctors," *Daily Dispatch* (Richmond), Oct. 20, 1875; Moore to unknown, Apr. 21, 1862, 707-VI-RG109; Moore to Polk, Jan. 29, 1864, *OR*, ser. 4, 3:59–60.

20. Gildersleeve, "History of Chimborazo Hospital"; Stout, "Best Models"; Stout, "Some Facts" (Sept. 1903): 517–19; Freeman, *Calendar of Confederate Papers*, 38.

21. *JCCSA*, 1:720–27, 5:288–90.

22. "Hospital Management," *Daily Richmond Examiner*, Aug. 27, 1862; Benjamin, "Regulations for the Care and Transportation of the Sick in the Army of the Potomac," ibid., Nov. 20, 1861.

23. Crocker, "Army Intelligence Office"; SO 173(32), July 24, 1864, 18-I-RG109; Stout, "Some Facts" (Oct. 1903): 570–71; Trans-Mississippi Department, GO 53, Nov. 12, 1863, *OR*, ser. 1, 22(2):1067–68.

24. "Report of the Select Committee on Hospitals," *Daily Richmond Enquirer*, Sept. 29, 1862; Act of Sept. 27, 1862, chap. 17, Cong. C.S.A. Stat. 63; GO 95, Nov. 25, 1862, 2-I-RG109; Warren, "Report of the Surgeon General," *Daily Progress* (Raleigh), Dec. 1, 2, 1864.

25. "Local Matters," *Daily Dispatch* (Richmond), Oct. 13, 1862; Carrington to Moore, Apr. 14, 1863, file for Carrington, microfilm M331(49); "Time of Closure of Hospls—Richmond," n.d., 151-VI-RG109.

26. Moore to Carrington, Feb. 2, 1863, 740(1)-VI-RG109; Carrington to Hines, Feb. 16, 1863, 416-VI-RG109; Carrington to Tompkins, June 15, 1864, 364-VI-RG109.

27. Warren, "Report of the Surgeon General," *Daily Progress* (Raleigh), Dec. 1, 2, 1864; Koonce, *Doctor to the Front*, 36; Wood, "Otis Frederick Manson"; Wood, "Surgeon General S. P. Moore"; Munson, *Confederate Incognito*; Long Grabs [Murdoch John McSween], "For the Observer," *Fayetteville (NC) Observer*, Nov. 6, 1862; "Office-Holders—Who Are They?" *Weekly Standard* (Raleigh), Mar. 11, 1863; Hilde, *Worth a Dozen Men*, 21.

28. Moore to James A. Seddon, Feb. 24, 1864, *OR*, ser. 1, 33:1196–98.

29. Synopsis of Consolidated Reports, 151-VI-RG109; Carrington to Moore, May 24, June 2, 1864, 364-VI-RG109; Moore to Carrington, June 2, 1864, 741(2)-VI-RG109.

30. Sorrel, circular, Aug. 1, 1862, 414½-VI-RG109; *JCCSA*, 6:282, 760. According to Thomas Fanning Wood, Surgeon Otis Manson gave the name "Moore Hospital" to the Richmond hospital he began directing in the spring of 1862 to honor the surgeon general. That, said Wood, displeased Moore, who preferred to have his name attached to a large pavilion hospital, so he had all of Richmond's hospitals numbered. Moore Hospital became General Hospital No. 24. Koonce, *Doctor to the Front*, 32, 199n2.

31. Carrington to Moore, Apr. 14, 1863, file for Carrington, microfilm M331 (49); Carrington to Moore, Feb. 13, 1864, and Moore to Davis, Feb. 15, 1864, in Jefferson Davis, "Message of the President," Feb. 16, 1864, https://archive.org/details/reportofapportio00conf/page/n1 (accessed Aug. 9, 2019); Moore to Thomas H. Williams, 739(2)-VI-RG109.

32. "Hospitals," *Daily Richmond Examiner*, Mar. 31, 1863; *JCCSA*, 3:216.

33. Jones, "Investigations upon the Nature," 153–54, 469; Moore, circular, July 6, 1863, Boston Athenaeum, http://catalog.bostonathenaeum.org/vwebv /holdingsInfo?bibId=325822 (accessed Sept. 8, 2018); Moore to Williams, Oct. 20, 1862, 739(2)-VI-RG109.

34. Welsh, *Two Confederate Hospitals*, 51; Gaillard, "In Memoriam"; Samuel H. Stout, Circular No. 38, Sept. 6, 1864, file for Bolling A. Pope, microfilm M331(200); Frank Hawthorn to Moore, Jan. 13, 1865, file for Hawthorn, microfilm M331(122); Carrington to John J. Gravatt, May 19, 1864, 337-VI-RG109; Carrington to William M. Gardner, Feb. 12, 1865, and Carrington to James B. Read, Feb. 18, 1865, 364-VI-RG109.

35. Carrington to Moore, June 16, 1864, and Carrington to William C. Nichols, Mar. 27, 1865, 364-VI-RG109.

36. Petition of Dental Surgeons, Dec. 29, 1863, entry 175, RG 109; Burton to William Porcher Miles, Jan. 5, 1864, and Moore to Carrington, Feb. 23, June 23, 1864, file for Burton, microfilm M331(42); Burton, "Dental Surgery."

37. Moore, circular, Feb. 6, 1865, 741(1)-VI-RG109; Stout, "Dental Surgeons"; Covey, "Interdental Splint"; Carrington to Moore, Feb. 20, 1865, and Carrington to Richmond and Petersburg surgeons, Feb. 20, 1865, 364-VI-RG109. After the war Bean formed a dental partnership with Asa H. Balderston, who had been on a wartime mission to buy medical supplies in the North (see chapter 7).

38. Carrington to James B. Gaston, Alexander G. Lane, Francis W. Hancock, and James B. McCaw, Feb. 4, 1865, 364-VI-RG109; William Duncan to Gaston, Mar. 30, 1865, file for Duncan, microfilm M331(81).

39. Act of May 1, 1863, chap. 86, Cong. C.S.A. Stat. 162; Hilde, *Worth a Dozen Men*, 124–30.

40. "Principle Hospitals in the Confederate States," "Army Medical Intelligence" (Sept., Oct. 1864).

41. Moore to William P. Miles, Dec. 14, 1861, entry UD 176A, RG 109; Moore, "Confederate Doctors," *Daily Dispatch* (Richmond), Oct. 20, 1875.

10. Prison Hospitals

1. Sanders, *While in the Hands of the Enemy*, 127–28; Act of May 21, 1861, chap. 59, Prov. Cong. C.S.A. Stat. 154; Walter Preston, "Report of the Committee on Quartermaster's and Commissary Departments," Feb. 13, 1864, *OR*, ser. 2, 6:950–52; Act of Feb. 17, 1864, chap. 47, Cong. C.S.A. Stat. 184.

2. SO 78(8), June 11, 1861, 6-I-RG109; Leroy P. Walker to J. Randolph Tucker and James Lyons, Aug. 30, 1861, *OR*, ser. 2, 2:1374; SO 129(16), June 3, 1864, 17-I-RG109; SO 175(48), July 26, 1864, 18-I-RG109; GO 84, Nov. 21, 1864, 4-I-RG109; Sanders, *While in the Hands of the Enemy*, 297–309.

3. GO 159, Dec. 4, 1863, 3-I-RG109; Moore, "Confederate Doctors," *Daily Dispatch* (Richmond), Oct. 20, 1875; Carrington to George W. Semple, July 12, 1864, 364-VI-RG109; SO 60(10), Mar. 12, 1863, 207-I-RG109.

4. Winder to Moore, Jan. 3, 1865, *OR*, ser. 2, 8:19.

5. Sanders, *While in the Hands of the Enemy*, 2–4, 122, 126–27; Thompson, "Treatment of Prisoners." Charles Sanders (*While in the Hands of the Enemy*) and William Hesseltine (*Civil War Prisons*) provide excellent descriptions and analyses of how POW management evolved throughout the war.

6. Moore to Walker, Aug. 1, 1861, *OR*, ser. 2, 3:698.

7. Moore to Walker, Aug. 1, 1861, *OR*, ser. 2, 3:700–701; Futch, *History of Andersonville Prison*, 119–29.

8. Dodge to Randolph, June 21, 1862, with endorsements, *OR*, ser. 2, 4:782–83; "The Seaman's Bethel," *Daily Dispatch* (Richmond), July 1, 1862.

9. Carrington to E. S. Gaillard, Oct. 3, 1862, file for Carrington, microfilm M331(49).

10. Moore to Seddon, July 30, 1863, *OR*, ser. 2, 6:181.

11. Sanders, *While in the Hands of the Enemy*, 163; Act of May 21, 1861, chap. 59, Prov. Cong. C.S.A. Stat. 154; Walter Preston, "Report of the Committee on Quartermaster's and Commissary Departments," Feb. 13, 1864, *OR*, ser. 2, 6:950–52; Preston to Seddon, Jan. 8, 1864, with enclosure, ibid., 821–22; Jones, *Rebel War Clerk's Diary*, 2:8.

12. Carrington to Winder, Mar. 23, 1864, with enclosures and endorsements, *OR*, ser. 2, 6:1084–90; "Gen. Morgan's Visit to Libby Prison," *Daily Richmond Enquirer*, Jan. 11, 1864; George W. Brent and Tobias G. Richardson to Braxton Bragg, Mar. 14, 1864, with enclosures and endorsements, *OR*, ser. 2, 6:1048–51.

13. Richardson to Bragg, Apr. 11, 1864, *OR*, ser. 2, 7:38–39.

14. Sanders, *While in the Hands of the Enemy*, 297–309.

15. Hesseltine, *Civil War Prisons*, 245–46; Futch, *History of Andersonville*, 120.

16. "Andersonville: Beginning of the Trial of Henry Wirz for the Murder of Union Soldiers," *New York World*, Aug. 22, 1865; "Trial of Henry Wirz: The First Day's Proceedings," *Daily National Intelligencer* (Washington, DC), Aug. 22, 1865; Chipman, *Horrors of Andersonville*, 12–18; *Trial of Henry Wirz*, 3–8, 615–18; "The Wirz Trial—Alleged Implication of Other Confederates," *Baltimore Sun*, Oct. 8, 1865; "Witness for Wirz," *Evening*

Star (Washington, DC), Oct. 11, 1865. Chipman's 1891 account of the trial erroneously included Jefferson Davis, but not Lucius B. Northrop, as a coconspirator in the original conspiracy charge. Chipman, *Horrors of Andersonville*, 13.

17. *Trial of Henry Wirz*, 805–8; Chipman, *Horrors of Andersonville*, 12–18; Dorris, *Pardon and Amnesty*, 313–16; Military Command of North Carolina, GO 35, Aug. 30, 1866, *OR*, ser. 2, 8:956–60; Adjutant General's Office, General Court-Martial Orders No. 153, June 8, 1866, ibid., 926–28.

18. *Trial of Henry Wirz*, 759–61; Jones, "Investigations upon the Diseases," 471–82; White to Daniel T. Chandler, Aug. 2, 1864, with endorsement, *OR*, ser. 2, 7:524–26.

19. Jones, "Investigations upon the Diseases," 471–82; Inquiries upon Hospital Gangrene, 226-IX-RG109.

20. Newton, "My Recollections," 488.

21. Schade, "Treatment of Federal Prisoners and Rebel Witnesses," *Daily National Intelligencer* (Washington, DC), Sept. 7, 1868.

22. Sanders, *While in the Hands of the Enemy*, 297–309; Carrington to Winder, Mar. 23, 1864, *OR*, ser. 2, 6:1084–90.

23. Jones, "Investigations upon the Diseases," 642–55.

24. Jones, "Investigations upon the Diseases," 614–15.

25. Jones, "Investigations upon the Diseases," 642–55; Invoices for H. H. Clayton, Mar. 24, 1865, and J. S. Dillard, Apr. 3, 1865, 630-VI-RG109; Invoice for R. R. Stevenson, Sept. 5, 1864, 632-VI-RG109; *Trial of Henry Wirz*, 28, 334; Hasegawa, "Quinine Substitutes." Acetic and citric acids, which were erroneously thought to be of benefit in scurvy, were also sent to Andersonville by the medical purveyor at Macon.

26. Ould, "Statement of Robert Ould, Esq.," *Daily National Intelligencer* (Washington, DC), Aug. 20, 1868; *Trial of Henry Wirz*, 334.

27. Jones, "Investigations upon the Diseases," 475; Gillett, *Army Medical Department*, 183–84.

28. Abraham Lincoln, proclamation, Dec. 8, 1863, 13 Stat. 737 (1866); Andrew Johnson, proclamation, May 29, 1865, 13 Stat. 758 (1866); File for Moore, microfilm M1003(65), RG 94; File for Brewer, microfilm M1003(57), ibid.

11. Striving for Quality in Medical Personnel

1. Wellington [pseud.], "Letter from the Army," *Daily Constitutionalist* (Augusta, GA), Sept. 14, 25, 1861; Army Surgeon, "'Iota' and 'The Army Surgeons,'" *Macon (GA) Daily Telegraph*, Dec. 20, 1862; Wailes, "Case of Field Surgery."

2. Wellington [pseud.], "Letter from the Army," *Daily Constitutionalist* (Augusta, GA), Sept. 14, 25, 1861; "The Medical Staff," *Daily Dispatch* (Richmond), Nov. 2, 1861.

3. War Department (Confederate), *Regulations for the Medical Department* (1861), 10–11; War Department (US), *Regulations for the Medical Department*, 14. The war did not last long enough for assistant surgeons in the regular army to serve for five years, but two—Andrew J. Foard and Richard Potts—were promoted to surgeon to fill vacancies caused by the promotion of Moore to surgeon general and the death of Surgeon Elisha P. Langworthy. Register of Regular Army Appointments, 88-I-RG109; *JCCSA*, 2:387.

4. Act of Mar. 6, 1861, chap. 26, § 9, Prov. Cong. C.S.A. Stat. 45, 46; Act of Mar. 6, 1861, chap. 29, § 10, Prov. Cong. C.S.A. Stat. 47, 48; SO 143(12), Sept. 4, 1861, 6-I-RG109; Brodie to Lorenzo Thomas, May 2, 1861, letter B197, microfilm M619(4), RG 94; Southgate to Thomas Lawson, Jan. 18, 1856, with endorsements, letter S44, microfilm M567(547), ibid.; "An Important Step Forward," *Charleston (SC) Mercury*, Sept. 11, 1861; Surgeon General's Office, notice of Sept. 27, 1861, ibid., Oct. 2, 1861.

5. Moore to Samuel Cooper, Mar. 3 (files S381 and S382), Mar. 6 (file S380), Mar. 13 (file S442), and Apr. 1 (file S576), 1862, microfilm M474(46); Moore to Cooper, Jan. 9 (file S31), Jan. 15 (file S69), and Feb. 5 (file S194), 1862, microfilm M474(45); J. C. Nott, "Army Surgeons," *Mobile Register and Advertiser*, Feb. 26, 1862; SO 84(31), Apr. 12, 1862, 213-I-RG109; SO 228(19), Sept. 30, 1862, SO 292(14), Dec. 13, 1862, and SO 295(10), Dec. 17, 1862, 206-I-RG109; Confidential instructions, Chattanooga, Mar. 21, 1863, box 2G407, Stout Papers, Dolph Briscoe Center for American History; SO 11(21), Jan. 14, 1863, 12-I-RG109; "Appendix: Medical Officers."

6. Guild to Moore, Oct. 25, Nov. 10, 1862, 641-VI-RG109; SO 266(16), Nov. 13, 1862, 11-I-RG109.

7. Bozeman to Thomas H. Williams, Oct. 6, 1861, file for Bozeman, microfilm M331(29).

8. "Army Medical Board."

9. "Letter from Norfolk," *Richmond Enquirer*, Sept. 27, 1861.

10. Coffin to Davis, Oct. 21, 1861, with endorsement, letter 7268, microfilm M437(14).

11. Gaston, "Personal and Surgical Reminiscences," 164–65.

12. "The Medical Staff," *Charleston (SC) Daily Courier*, Mar. 5, 1862; "The Army Medical Board," *Daily Richmond Examiner*, Oct. 19, 1861.

13. Samuel Preston Moore, confidential instructions, Knoxville, Oct. 1, 1862, and confidential instructions, Chattanooga, Mar. 21, 1863, box 2G407,

Stout Papers, Dolph Briscoe Center for American History; Moore, "Instructions to Applicants for Appointment in the Medical Department," n.d., 739(2)-VI-RG109; Roberts, "Organization and Personnel of the Medical Department," 352; Koonce, *Doctor to the Front*, 41–42.

14. Moore, "Instructions to Assistant Surgeons Applying for Promotion in the Medical Department," n.d., 739(2)-VI-RG109; Guild to Moore, Oct. 25, 1862, 641-VI-RG109; SO 298(21), Dec. 20, 1862, 11-I-RG109.

15. Moore, "Instructions to Applicants for Appointment in the Medical Department," n.d., and "Instructions to Assistant Surgeons Applying for Promotion in the Medical Department," n.d., 739(2)-VI-RG109; Moore, confidential instructions, Knoxville, Oct. 1, 1862, and confidential instructions, Chattanooga, Mar. 21, 1863, box 2G407, Stout Papers, Dolph Briscoe Center for American History; Williams, *Rebel Brothers*, 15–85; Koonce, *Doctor to the Front*, 38–42; SO 41(4), Feb. 18, 1863, 207-I-RG109; MCV, advertisement, *Daily Richmond Examiner*, Sept. 11, 1861.

16. Moore to AIGO, Feb. 5, 1862, file S194, microfilm M474(45); SO 4(10), Jan. 6, 1862, 8-I-RG109; Hambrecht, "J. J. Chisolm."

17. Bollet, *Civil War Medicine*, 57–60; Warner, *Therapeutic Perspective*, 169–75; Park to Confederate Senate, Oct. 7, 1862, entry 175, RG 109.

18. Scrutator [pseud.], "The Army Medical Board of Examination Convened at Charleston, S.C.," *Daily Richmond Examiner*, Mar. 18, 1862; Koste, "Medical School for a Nation," 31; Simons, "To the Medical Fraternity of Charleston," *Charleston (SC) Daily Courier*, Apr. 1, 1862; Simons to Samuel Cooper, Feb. 21, 1862, letter S329, and Simons to Moore, Mar. 13, 1862, letter S494, microfilm M474(45); Warren, *Doctor's Experiences*, 287–88; SO 10(9), Jan. 13, 1862, 213-I-RG109; "Appendix: Medical Officers"; Pember, *Southern Woman's Story*, 90; Iota [pseud.], "The Army Surgeons," *Macon (GA) Daily Telegraph*, Dec. 12, 1862; Nott, "Army Surgeons," *Mobile Register and Advertiser*, Feb. 26, 1862.

19. Monteiro, *War Reminiscences*, 23–26; Daniel, *Recollections of a Rebel Surgeon*, 39–40; Baruch, "An Ex-Confederate's Experiences," *Long Branch (NJ) Daily Record*, Oct. 5, 1915, 11–12.

20. Benjamin to Jefferson Davis, Dec. [14?], 1861, *OR*, ser. 4, 1:794; Moore, "Confederate Doctors," *Daily Dispatch* (Richmond), Oct. 20, 1875; Roberts, "Organization and Personnel of the Medical Department," 352; "Letter from Norfolk," *Richmond Enquirer*, Sept. 27, 1861.

21. Moore, circular, Aug. 15, 1863, *OR*, ser. 4, 2:723.

22. Moore to William A. Carrington, Apr. 6, 1863; 740(1)-VI-RG109; Moore, circular, Dec. 15, 1863, 740(2)-VI-RG109; Moore, circular, Mar. 24, 1863, 739(1)-VI-RG109.

23. War Department (Confederate), *Regulations for the Medical Department* (1862), 14; Moore, circular, Aug. 27, 1863, 557-VI-RG109.

24. Carrington, circular, Sept. 3, 1863, SO 9, Sept. 9, 1863, and Carrington to Courtenay J. Clark, Sept. 8, 1863, 557-VI-RG109; Sites to George S. Barnsley, Sept. 6, 1863, *George Scarborough Barnsley Papers.*

25. Koste, "Medical School for a Nation"; Rothstein, *American Medical Schools*, 49; Slawson, "Medical Training"; Moore, "Confederate Doctors," *Daily Dispatch* (Richmond), Oct. 20, 1875.

26. "Necrology: James T. Meek"; L. S. Joynes, MCV Statement of Graduates, 1863–64, Sanger Historical Files, Tompkins-McCaw Library; Meek to Carrington, July 23, 1863, file for Meek, microfilm M331(175); R. F. Baldwin to Thomas H. Williams, Nov. 23, 1862, file for Trueheart, microfilm M331(251).

27. Joynes, MCV Statement of Graduates, 1861–62, 1863–64, Sanger Historical Files, Tompkins-McCaw Library.

12. Adding to Medical Knowledge

1. Campbell, "Hunterian Ligation," 201; Talley to E. B. Turnipseed, Nov. 6, 1861, "Letter Book of Medical Director's Office," Wessels Library; Gross, "Manual of Military Surgery"; Gross, *Manual of Military Surgery.*

2. Macleod, *Notes on the Surgery*; "New Publication," *Daily Dispatch* (Richmond), June 18, 1862; J. W. Randolph, advertisement, *Richmond Whig*, June 19, 1862.

3. Chisolm, *Manual of Military Surgery*, 1st, 2nd, and 3rd eds.; Evans & Cogswell, advertisement, *Camden (SC) Daily Journal*, July 21, 1864; Evans & Cogswell to William Porcher Miles, Dec. 1, 1864, letter E759, microfilm M474(110); Warren, *Epitome of Practical Surgery*; Warren, *Doctor's Experiences*, 306–7; Warren to Moore, Sept. 9, 1862, file for Warren, microfilm M331(260); Abernathy, "Manual of Military Surgery," 675; Newton, "My Recollections," 477.

4. Moore, "Confederate Doctors," *Daily Dispatch* (Richmond), Oct. 20, 1875; "The Medical and Surgical Journal," *Southern Illustrated News* (Richmond), Nov. 7, 1863.

5. *Manual of Military Surgery*; *Medical and Surgical History*, 2(2):810n2; "The Medical and Surgical Journal," *Southern Illustrated News* (Richmond), Nov. 7, 1863; Wright, "Effects of Hunterian Method"; Campbell, "Hunterian Ligation," 201–2; Watson, *Physicians and Surgeons*, 99; Abernathy, "Manual of Military Surgery"; A. J. Foard to Moore, Apr. 18, 1864, 748-VI-RG109. The book appears to have been first available in early 1864. See "Recent Publications," *Richmond Whig and Public Advertiser*, Feb. 5, 1864.

6. Porcher, *Resources*; *General Directions*; Moore, circular, Apr. 2, 1862, *OR*, ser. 4, 1:1041; Surgeon General's Office, order, May 27, 1862, and Moore to Porcher, June 10, 1862, Wickham Family Papers, Virginia Historical Society.

7. "Resources of Our Forests," *Charleston (SC) Daily Courier*, Jan. 6, 1863; Carrington to Moore, Apr. 27, 1863, 416-VI-RG109.

8. "Resources of the Southern Fields and Forests," *Charleston (SC) Daily Courier*, May 7, 1863; Hasegawa, "Southern Resources"; Guerard, "Our Botanical Resources," *Charleston (SC) Daily Courier*, Oct. 31, 1864; Evans & Cogswell, invoice, Mar. 18, 1863, microfilm M346(288); Porcher, *Resources* (Richmond ed. only), ii; West & Johnston, advertisement, *Southern Illustrated News*, May 2, 1863, 8; S. G. Courtenay's, advertisement, *Charleston (SC) Daily Courier*, Jan. 19, 1863; Wedderburn & Alfriend, advertisement, *Sentinel* (Richmond), Apr. 2, 1864; *Standard Supply Table*; *General Directions*.

9. Moore, "Confederate Doctors," *Daily Dispatch* (Richmond), Oct. 20, 1875; "Resources of Our Fields and Forests," *Richmond Whig and Public Advertiser*, Apr. 28, 1863; "Resources of Our Fields and Forests," *Charleston (SC) Mercury*, Apr. 29, 1863; "Resources of the Southern Fields and Forests," *Wilmington (NC) Journal*, Apr. 30, 1863; "Resources of Our Fields and Forests," *Daily Constitutionalist* (Augusta, GA), May 1, 1863; "Resources of Our Fields and Forests," *Wilmington (NC) Journal*, May 7, 1863. Given that *Resources* became available two years before the surrender of the Army of Northern Virginia, the estimate of one historian that the book "saved the Confederacy for two years at least" seems exaggerated. James Henry Rice Jr., "Paladins of South Carolina: Francis Peyre Porcher," *State* (Columbia, SC), Sept. 14, 1924. For more discussion of the value of Porcher's book, see Hasegawa, "Southern Resources."

10. "Association of Army and Navy Surgeons"; Freeman, *Calendar of Confederate Papers*, 33–43.

11. Freeman, *Calendar of Confederate Papers*, 33–43; *Medical and Surgical History*, 2(1):xxi–xxii; Koonce, *Doctor to the Front*, 50; Lane, "Winder Hospital," 39–40.

12. Moore, circular, June 25, 1862, 739(1)-VI-RG109.

13. Moore, circular, Apr. 25, 1863, 740(1)-VI-RG109.

14. Hicks, "Scabrous Matters"; Moore to William A Carrington, June 15, 1863; 740(1)-VI-RG109; Moore to Edward A. Flewellen, July 31, 1863, 748-VI-RG109.

15. Moore to Williams, Jan. 7, 1862, 739(1)-VI-RG109; Williams to John B. Fontaine, Jan. 30, 1862, and Williams to Moore, Feb. 8, 1862, 460-VI-RG109; Robert J. Breckinridge to Hunter Holmes McGuire, Feb. 1, 1863,

641-VI-RG109; Moore to Flewellen, July 31, 1863, 748-VI-RG109; Moore, circular, Oct. 16, 1863, National Library of Medicine, http://resource.nlm.nih.gov/101645108 (accessed Aug. 11, 2019); Moore, circular, May 13, 1862, 739(1)-VI-RG109.

16. "A Medical and Surgical Journal," *Southern Illustrated News* (Richmond), Oct. 24, 1863; "A Medical and Surgical Journal Again," ibid., Oct. 31, 1863; "The Medical and Surgical Journal," ibid., Nov. 7, 1863.

17. "Revival of Medical Journalism"; Ayres & Wade, circular and prospectus, *Southern Illustrated News* (Richmond), Jan. 30, 1864, 4; "Salutatory"; "Confederate States Medical and Surgical Journal," *Southern Illustrated News* (Richmond), Jan. 9, 1864; "Dr. James B. McCaw"; "Obituary Record: Dr. William Middleton Michel."

18. "Amputation, Disarticulation and Resection"; "Conservative Surgery"; Sorrel, "Gun-Shot Wounds"; "Prospect before Us"; "To the Reader."

19. Warren, *Epitome of Practical Surgery*, ii; Chisolm, *Manual of Military Surgery*, 3rd ed., vii; Newton, "My Recollections," 484; Moore, "Confederate Doctors," *Daily Dispatch* (Richmond), Oct. 20, 1875.

20. Evans & Cogswell to William Porcher Miles, Dec. 1, 1864, letter E759, microfilm M474(110).

13. Examining for Disability

1. Act of Apr. 16, 1862, chap. 30, Cong. C.S.A. Stat. 29; GO 30, Apr. 28, 1862, 2-I-RG109.

2. GO 32, Apr. 30, 1862, 2-I-RG109; War Department (Confederate), *Regulations for the Medical Department* (1862), 11.

3. John Dunwody, notice, *Daily Chronicle & Sentinel* (Augusta, GA), July 1, 1862; Moore, circular, July 3, 1862, *OR*, ser. 4, 2:2; Letcher, message to Virginia Senate and House of Delegates, Mar. 25, 1862, ibid., 1:1021–22.

4. Dunwoody [*sic*], "Instructions to Enrolling Officers," *Daily Chronicle & Sentinel* (Augusta, GA), June 30 1862; Dunwoody [*sic*], "New Conscription Orders," ibid., Aug. 5, 1862. Dunwody's name was often misspelled as "Dunwoody."

5. "Despotic," *Daily Constitutionalist* (Augusta, GA), Aug. 3, 1862; "Abuse of the Conscript Law," ibid., Aug. 15, 1862; GO 58, Aug. 14, 1862, 2-I-RG109; GO 65(5), Sept. 9, 1862, 2-I-RG109.

6. Act of Oct. 11, 1862, chap. 41, Cong. C.S.A. Stat. 75; GO 82(6), Nov. 3, 1862, and GO 101(1), Dec. 9, 1862, 2-I-RG109.

7. Moore to Samuel Cooper, Nov. 25, 1862, with endorsements, file S2759, microfilm M474(48); Alexander and Beringer, *Anatomy of the Confederate*

Congress, 12; SO 294(14, 15), Dec. 16, 1862, SO 296(3, 4), Dec. 18, 1862, and SO 303(6), Dec. 27, 1862, 11-I-RG109; SO 4(7, 10, 11), Jan. 6, 1863, 12-I-RG109.

8. GO 22, Feb. 23, 1863, 3-I-RG109; GO 11(1), Feb. 1, 1864, 4-I-RG109.

9. Cooper, third enclosure, in John S. Preston to Davis, Nov. 28, 1864, *OR*, ser. 4, 3:854–63.

10. Walter to J. W. C. Watson, Dec. 29, 1864, *OR*, ser. 4, 3:976–79.

11. GO 77, Oct. 8, 1864, 4-I-RG109; SO 257(4), Oct. 28, 1864, 19-I-RG109; Moore to James L. Kemper, Oct. 20, 1864, file S5017, microfilm M474(144); Moore to James A. Seddon, Dec. 13, 1864, file M4492, microfilm M474(132).

12. Ramsdell, *Laws and Joint Resolutions*, 86–88, 150–51; Richardson, *Compilation of the Messages and Papers*, 542–43; Cooper, third enclosure, in John S. Preston to Davis, Nov. 28, 1864, *OR*, ser. 4, 3:854–63.

13. GO 10(4–9), Mar. 17, 1865, *OR*, ser. 4, 3:1152–53.

14. AIGO, *Regulations Published for Guidance of the Army*, 1; SO 17, Nov. 7, 1861, 1-I-RG109; *JCCSA*, 5:288–90; GO 9(12), June 25, 1861, 1-I-RG109.

15. Davis, *Message of the President*, with enclosures.

16. "The Examining Board—The Provost Department of Richmond," *Daily Richmond Examiner*, Aug. 26, 1862; "Ill Treatment of Soldiers in Hospitals," *Fayetteville (NC) Observer*, Aug. 25, 1862.

17. Davis, *Message of the President*, with enclosures; "The Confederate Congress," *Daily Richmond Examiner*, Sept. 4, 5, 1862; *JCCSA*, 5:347. It is unclear whether Strickland was referring to the original Richmond board only or also to those at Chimborazo and Winder Hospitals.

18. "General Hospital at Camp Winder," *Richmond Whig and Public Advertiser*, Sept. 12, 1862.

19. "The Confederate Congress," *Daily Richmond Examiner*, Sept. 20, 1862; Georgian [pseud.], letter, *Daily Richmond Examiner*, Sept. 23, 1862; Davis, *Message of the President*, with enclosures; Mitchell, *Charge to the Graduates*, 13; *Catalogue of the Graduates*, 101, 108.

20. "Report of the Select Committee on Hospitals," *Daily Richmond Enquirer*, Sept. 29, 1862; Act of May 1, 1863, chap. 49, Cong. C.S.A. Stat. 153.

21. GO 72(4, 5), Sept. 29, 1862, and GO 107(1, 2), Dec. 17, 1862, 2-I-RG109; GO 51, Apr. 29, 1863, 3-I-RG109.

22. Guild to Moore, Jan. 14, 1863, and Guild to Walter H. Taylor, Jan. 5, 1863, 641-VI-RG109; *JCCSA*, 5:288–90; Carrington to McCaw, June 3, 1864, 709-VI-RG109.

23. Act of May 1, 1863, chap. 49, Cong. C.S.A. Stat. 153; GO 69, May 28, 1863, and GO 141, Oct. 20, 1863, 3-I-RG109; GO 11, Feb. 1, 1864, and GO 25,

Feb. 29, 1864, 4-I-RG109; Act of Feb. 17, 1864, chap. 48, Cong. C.S.A. Stat. 194.

24. Carrington to Moore, June 1, 1864, 364-VI-RG109.

25. Carrington to Moore, June 1, 1864, 364-VI-RG109; Guild to Taylor, Jan. 27, 1865, 642-VI-RG109.

26. Act of Feb. 17, 1864, chap. 55, Cong. C.S.A. Stat. 203; GO 34, Mar. 16, 1864, 4-I-RG109; Ramsdell, *Laws and Joint Resolutions*, 27–28.

27. Moore, Circular No. 6, Mar. 24, 1864, with endorsements, file B972, microfilm M474(94).

14. War's End and Beyond

1. Moore to Samuel Cooper, Apr. 1, 1865, file M727, microfilm M474(160).

2. Mallory, "Last Days of the Confederate Government"; Parker, *Recollections of a Naval Officer*, 372–96; "Captured Documents," *Commercial Bulletin* (Richmond), May 17, 1865; Moore, "Confederate Doctors," *Daily Dispatch* (Richmond), Oct. 20, 1875.

3. Moore to Cooper, Apr. 6, 1865, file M657, and Moore to Cooper, Apr. 26, 1865 (two letters), files M663 and M664, microfilm M474(160); Chisolm to Moore, Apr. 19 (four letters), Feb. 17, 1865, collection of Jonathan O'Neal, MD; Chisolm to Moore, Feb. 17, 1865, box 83 (55), R. A. Brock Collection and Papers, Huntington Library; Moore to Chisolm, Apr. 21, 25, 26, 1865, collection of the J. J. Chisolm family; George S. Blackie, SO, July 23, 1864, file for Ray, microfilm M331(207).

4. Snipes to Judah Benjamin, Oct. 1861, file for Snipes, microfilm M346(961); Return of Civil and Military Officers, file 3055, entry 183, RG 109; Moore to Andrew Johnson, June 23, 1865, and Moore, oath, June 22, 1865, file for Moore, microfilm M1003(65), RG 94; Williams, oath, June 22, 1865, file for Williams, microfilm M1003(30), ibid.; CSR for Williams, microfilm M331(259).

5. CSR for Smith, microfilm M331(228); Williams, oath, June 22, 1865, file for Williams, microfilm M1003(30), RG 94; CSR for Williams, microfilm M331(259); CSR for Sorrel, file for Sorrell [*sic*], microfilm M331(223); CSR for Baer, file for Bair [*sic*], microfilm M331(12); Brewer to Andrew Johnson, May 11, 1865, file for Brewer, microfilm M1003(57), RG 94; CSR for Brewer, microfilm M331(32).

6. Carrington to Andrew Johnson, July 14, 1865, file for Carrington, microfilm M1003(58), RG 94; CSR for Johns, microfilm M331(140).

7. "Death of a South Carolinian Abroad," *Charleston (SC) Daily News*, Sept. 25, 1872; Elzas, *Jews of South Carolina*, 271–73; Wiernik, *History of the Jews*

in America, 162; Bertram Jonas, "Surgeon Soldier of the Mexican War," *American Jewish Outlook* (Pittsburgh), May 27, 1938; Burns, "David Camden De Leon."

8. Smith obituary, *Daily Dispatch* (Richmond), Mar. 25, 1879; "Statue to a Forgotten Hero," *Times Dispatch* (Richmond), May 15, 1910.

9. "Dr. Samuel P. Moore," *Richmond Dispatch*, June 1, 1889; Lewis, "Samuel Preston Moore"; *Sheriff & Chataigne's Richmond City Directory*, 156; *Sheriff & Co.'s Richmond City Directory*, 143; Moore, "Confederate Doctors," *Daily Dispatch* (Richmond), Oct. 20, 1875. There was considerable inconsistency in how the name of the Association of Medical Officers of the Confederate States Army and Navy was rendered in various publications. The version used here is close to, if not exactly, the official name. Moore's 1875 address, appearing originally in Richmond's *Daily Dispatch* of October 20, 1875, became more widely available when reprinted thirty-four years later. Moore, "Address of the President".

10. "Description of the Model"; *Year Book, 1911–1912*, 23–24; Cunningham, *Doctors in Gray*; Bollet, *Civil War Medicine*, 15–16; Farr, "Samuel Preston Moore."

Conclusion

1. Faust, *This Republic of Suffering*, 250–65; *Medical and Surgical History*, 1(3):29–33.

2. Porcher, "Confederate Surgeons," 16–17; Gaillard, "Medical and Surgical Lessons," 715–16.

3. Chancellor, "Memoir of the Late Samuel Preston Moore," 636–37; Lewis, "Samuel Preston Moore," 385; "Dr. Samuel Preston Moore," *Richmond Dispatch*, June 1, 1889; Porcher, "Confederate Surgeons," 15; Collins, "System in the South," 517; Vandiver, *Ploughshares into Swords*.

4. Hambrecht, "J. J. Chisolm"; Chisolm, *Manual of Military Surgery*, 3rd ed., iii.

Bibliography

Archives

Dolph Briscoe Center for American History, University of Texas at Austin
    Samuel Hollingsworth Stout Papers
Huntington Library, San Marino, CA
    R. A. Brock Collection and Papers
National Archives and Records Administration, Washington, DC (NARA)
    Record Group (RG) 94: Records of the Adjutant General's Office,
    1780s–1917
        Microfilm M567 and M619: Letters Received by the Office of the
        Adjutant General (Main Series)
        Microfilm M1003: Case Files of Applications from Former
        Confederates for Presidential Pardons ("Amnesty Papers")
    RG 109: War Department Collection of Confederate Records
        Chap. I: Adjutant and Inspector General's Department
            Vols. 1–4 and 203: General Orders, 1861–65
            Vols. 6, 8, 9, 11, 13–18, 204–8, 210, 213, and 218: Special
            Orders, 1861–64
            Vol. 35: Letters and Telegrams Sent, Mar.–Aug. 1861
            Vols. 45 and 46: Registers of Letters Received, 1861
            Vol. 54: Register of Letters Received, Jan.–Mar. 1863, N–Z
            Vol. 68: Register of Letters Received, Oct. 1864–Mar. 1865,
            G–M
            Vol. 88: Register of Regular Army Officers
            Vol. 119: Record of Appointment of Officers, 1861–62
            Vol. 128: Record of Appointment of Officers, 1864–65
        Chap. VI: Medical Department
            Vols. 6, 135, 566, and 628: Letters, Telegrams, Orders, and
            Circulars Received at Medical Purveyor's Office, Savannah
            and Macon, 1862–65
            Vol. 7: Orders and Circulars Received, Chimborazo Hospital
            No. 1, 1863–64
            Vol. 151: Statistical Reports of Hospitals in Virginia, 1862–64

Vol. 337: Letters Received and Sent, General Hospital No. 9, 1864–65

Vol. 364: Letters Sent and Received, Medical Director, Richmond, 1864–65

Vol. 367: Letters Sent, Medical Director's Office, Army of the Potomac, Sept. 1861–Jan. 1862

Vol. 414½: Letters, Orders, and Circulars Issued and Received; Lists of Deaths; and Lists of Patients Treated in Private Quarters, General Hospital No. 18, 1862–63

Vol. 416: Letters Sent and Received, Medical Director's Office, Richmond, 1862–63

Vol. 460: Letters Sent, Medical Director's Office, Army of the Potomac, Jan. 14-May 1862

Vol. 557: Reports of the Board for Examining Hospital Stewards, 1863–64

Vols. 572 and 627: Letters and Telegrams Sent from Medical Purveyor's Office, Savannah and Macon, 1862–64

Vol. 623: Account Book of the Macon Office, 1862–65

Vol. 629: Letters Sent, Medical Purveyor's Office, Western Department, 1863–65

Vols. 630 and 632: Invoices of Requisitions for Medical Supplies Made on the Depot of the Macon Office, 1864–65

Vol. 641: Letters Sent by the Medical Director's Office, Army of Northern Virginia, June 29, 1862–Aug. 29, 1863

Vols. 707–9: Letters Received and Sent, Chimborazo Hospital, 1861–64

Vols. 739–41: Letters, Orders, and Circulars Sent, Surgeon General's Office, 1861–65

Vol. 748: Letters, Orders, and Circulars Sent and Received, Medical Director's Office, Army of Tennessee, 1862–65

Vol. 750: Letters, Telegrams, Orders, and Circulars Issued and Received, Medical Purveyor's Office, Army of Tennessee, 1862–63

Chap. IX: Office of the Secretary of War

Vols. 87 and 88: War Department Payrolls, Jul. 1862–Mar. 1865

Vol. 226: Reports on Conditions at Andersonville Prison, 1864–65

Entry 60: Payrolls of Extra Duty Men, 1861–65

Entry 175: Memorials and Petitions, 1861–65

Entry UD 176A: Communications from the Confederate War Department to the Confederate Congress

Entry 183: Manuscripts, 1861–65

Entry 187: Papers of Lt. Col. John Withers, ca. 1840–60

Microfilm M311: Compiled Service Records of Confederate Soldiers Who Served in Organizations from the State of Alabama

Microfilm M324: Compiled Service Records of Confederate Soldiers Who Served in Organizations from the State of Virginia

Microfilm M331: Compiled Service Records of Confederate Generals and Staff Officers, and Nonregimental Enlisted Men

Microfilm M345: Union Provost Marshal's File of Papers Relating to Individual Civilians

Microfilm M346: Confederate Papers Relating to Citizens or Business Firms

Microfilm M437: Letters Received by the Confederate Secretary of War, 1861–65

Microfilm M474: Letters Received by the Confederate Adjutant and Inspector General, 1861–65

Microfilm M522: Letters Sent by the Confederate Secretary of War, 1861–65

Microfilm M627: Letters and Telegrams Sent by the Confederate Adjutant and Inspector General, 1861–65

Microfilm M935: Inspection Reports and Related Records Received by the Inspection Branch in the Confederate Adjutant and Inspector General's Office

Papers of Aaron Snowden Piggot, M.D., 1874–99

Tompkins-McCaw Library, Special Collections and Archives, Virginia Commonwealth University, Richmond

Sanger Historical Files

Virginia Historical Society, Richmond

Wickham Family Papers

Waring Historical Library, Medical University of South Carolina, Charleston

Francis Peyre Porcher Papers

Wessels Library, Newberry College, Newberry, SC

"Letter Book of Dr. J. J. Chisolm, Medical Purveyor, C.S.A., Columbia, S.C., May 24 to Nov. 14, 1862." Letterbooks of J. J. Chisolm.

Unpublished transcription by F. Terry Hambrecht. Copy of Microsoft Word file in author's possession.

"Letter Book of Medical Director's Office, Charleston, SC, Oct. 8, 1861, to Nov. 18, 1861, and the Medical Purveyor's Office, Charleston, SC, Nov. 19, 1861, to June 5, 1862." Letterbooks of J. J. Chisolm. Unpublished transcription by F. Terry Hambrecht. Copy of Microsoft Word file in author's possession.

Wilson Library, Southern Historical Collection, University of North Carolina at Chapel Hill

Augustus Coutanche Evans Papers, #2991-z

James King Hall Papers, #1563

Articles, Books, and Dissertations

Abernathy, J. C. "Manual of Military Surgery for the Army of the Confederate States." *Southern Practitioner* 24, no. 12 (Dec. 1902): 674–79.

Adams, Ephraim Douglass. *Great Britain and the American Civil War.* Vol. 1. Gloucester, MA: Peter Smith, 1957.

Addresses Delivered on the Occasion of the Dedication of the Hartford Hospital. Hartford, CT: Case, Lockwood, 1859.

Adjutant and Inspector General's Office. *Regulations Published for the Guidance of the Army.* Richmond, Aug. 1861. https://archive.org/details/followingregula 00conf/page/n1. Accessed Aug. 11, 2019.

Alexander, Thomas B., and Richard E. Beringer. *The Anatomy of the Confederate Congress.* Nashville: Vanderbilt University Press, 1972.

"Amputation, Disarticulation and Resection Statistics of the Confederate States Army." *Confederate States Medical and Surgical Journal* 1, no. 5 (May 1864): 77–78.

"Appendix: Medical Officers, Trans-Mississippi Department." In *Confederate Military History,* 10: 377–87. Atlanta: Confederate Publishing, 1899.

"Army Medical Board." *Southern Medical and Surgical Journal* 17, no. 19 (Oct. 1861): 825.

"Army Medical Intelligence." *Confederate States Medical and Surgical Journal* 1, no. 9 (Sept. 1864): 152; no. 10 (Oct. 1864): 176; no. 11 (Nov. 1864): 200.

"Association of Army and Navy Surgeons." *Confederate States Medical and Surgical Journal* 1, no. 1 (Jan. 1864): 13–16.

Barnwell, R. W., Jr., G. H. McMaster, M. La Borde, T. A. Lafar, G. W. Hicks, and E. E. Jackson. *Report of the South Carolina Hospital Aid Association in Virginia, 1861–1862.* Richmond: Macfarland & Fergusson, 1862.

Bartholomees, J. Boone, Jr. *Buff Facings and Gilt Buttons: Staff and Headquarters Operations in the Army of Northern Virginia, 1861–1865.* Columbia, SC: University of South Carolina Press, 1988.

Basler, Roy P. *The Collected Works of Abraham Lincoln.* Vol. 1. New Brunswick, NJ: Rutgers University Press, 1953.

Berlin, Jean V., ed. *A Confederate Nurse: The Diary of Ada W. Bacot, 1860–1863.* Columbia: University of South Carolina Press, 1994.

Biographical Review: This Volume Contains Biographical Sketches of Leading Citizens of Cumberland County, New Jersey. Boston: Biographical Review, 1896.

Blakey, Arch Fredric. *General John H. Winder, C.S.A.* Gainesville: University of Florida Press, 1990.

Blanton, Wyndham B. *Medicine in Virginia in the Nineteenth Century.* Richmond, VA: Garrett & Massie, 1933.

Bollet, Alfred Jay. *Civil War Medicine: Challenges and Triumphs.* Tucson: Galen, 2002.

Brock, Sarah Ann. *Richmond during the War.* New York: G. W. Carleton, 1867.

Buck, Alice Trueheart. "Founder of the First Confederate Hospital." *Confederate Veteran* 2, no. 5 (May 1894): 141.

Burns, Stanley B. "David Camden De Leon." *Judeo Medical Journal* 2 (Dec. 2001–Jan. 2002): 8.

Burton, W. Leigh. "Dental Surgery as Applied in the Armies of the Late Confederate States." *American Journal of Dental Science*, 3rd ser., vol. 1, no. 4 (Aug. 1867): 180–89.

Butler, Pierce. *Judah P. Benjamin.* Philadelphia: George W. Jacobs, 1907.

Calcutt, Rebecca Barbour. *Richmond's Wartime Hospitals.* Greta, LA: Pelican, 2005.

Campbell, Henry F. "The Hunterian Ligation of Arteries to Relieve and to Prevent Destructive Inflammation." *Southern Journal of the Medical Sciences* 1 (Aug. 1866): 201–18.

Capers, Henry D. *The Life and Times of C. G. Memminger.* Richmond: Everett Waddey, 1893.

Catalogue of the Alumni of the Medical Department of the University of Pennsylvania, 1765–1877. Philadelphia: Collins, 1877.

Catalogue of the Graduates and Officers of the Medical Department of the University of the City of New York. 3rd ed. New York: Douglas Taylor, 1890.

Chancellor, Charles W. "A Memoir of the Late Samuel Preston Moore, M.D., Surgeon General of the Confederate States Army." *Southern Practitioner* 25, no. 11 (Nov. 1903): 634–43.

Chandler, David G. *The Campaigns of Napoleon*. New York: Scribner, 1966.

Chipman, Norton P. *The Horrors of Andersonville Rebel Prison*. San Francisco: Bancroft, 1891.

Chisolm, J. Julian. *A Manual of Military Surgery for the Use of the Confederate Army*. 1st ed. Columbia, SC: Evans & Cogswell; Richmond: West & Johnston, 1861.

———. *A Manual of Military Surgery for the Use of the Confederate Army*. 2nd ed. Richmond: West & Johnston, 1862.

———. *A Manual of Military Surgery for the Use of the Confederate Army*. 3rd ed. Columbia, SC: Evans & Cogswell, 1864.

The City Intelligencer; or, Stranger's Guide. Richmond: Macfarlane & Fergusson, 1862.

Claiborne, John Herbert. *Seventy-Five Years in Old Virginia*. New York: Neale, 1904.

Cleland, Robert G. "Jefferson Davis and the Confederate Congress." *Southwestern Historical Quarterly* 19, no. 3 (Jan. 1916): 213–31.

Cole, W. H. "Manufacture and Consumption of Quinine in the United States." *Pharmaceutical Journal* 14 (July 1, 1854): 15–16.

Collins, Steven G. "System in the South: John W. Mallett, Josiah Gorgas, and Uniform Production at the Confederate Ordnance Department." *Technology and Culture* 40, no. 3 (July 1999): 517–44.

Collins, William H. *The Collins Family*. Quincy, IL: Volk, Jones, & McMein, 1897.

"Commercial Dependence of the South on the North." *De Bow's Southern and Western Review*, n.s., 2, no. 3 (Mar. 1852): 299–300.

"Conservative Surgery in Compound Fracture of Femur." *Confederate States Medical and Surgical Journal* 1, no. 6 (June 1864): 89–90.

Correspondence Concerning Claims against Great Britain. Vol. 7. Washington, DC: Government Printing Office, 1871.

Coulter, E. Merton. *The Confederate States of America, 1861–1865*. Baton Rouge: Louisiana State University Press, 1950.

Covey, Edward N. "The Interdental Splint." *Richmond Medical Journal* 1 (Feb. 1866): 81–91.

Crist, Lynda Lasswell, and Mary Seaton Dix, eds. *The Papers of Jefferson Davis*. Vol. 7, *1861*. Baton Rouge: Louisiana State University Press, 1992.

Crist, Lynda Lasswell, Kenneth H. Williams, and Peggy L. Dillard, eds. *The Papers of Jefferson Davis*. Vol. 10, *October 1863–August 1864*. Baton Rouge: Louisiana State University Press, 1999.

Crocker, W. A. "The Army Intelligence Office." *Confederate Veteran* 8, no. 3 (Mar. 1900): 118–19.

Cunningham, Horace Herndon. "Confederate General Hospitals: Establishment and Organization." *Journal of Southern History* 20, no. 3 (Aug. 1954): 376–94.

———. "The Confederate Medical Officer in the Field." *Bulletin of the New York Academy of Medicine* 34, no. 7 (July 1958): 461–88.

———. *Doctors in Gray: The Confederate Medical Service.* Baton Rouge: Louisiana State University Press, 1958.

———. *Field Medical Services at the Battles of Manassas (Bull Run).* Athens: University of Georgia Press, 1968.

———. "The Medical Service and Hospitals of the Southern Confederacy." PhD diss., University of North Carolina, 1952.

———. "Organization and Administration of the Confederate Medical Department." *North Carolina Historical Review* 31, no. 3 (July 1954): 385–409.

Daniel, F. E. *Recollections of a Rebel Surgeon (and Other Sketches); or, In the Doctor's Sappy Days.* Austin, TX: Von Boeckmann, Schutze, 1899.

Dauber, Leonard G. "David Camden DeLeon, M.D.: Patriot or Traitor." *New York State Journal of Medicine* 70, no. 23 (Dec. 1, 1970): 2927–33.

Davis, Jefferson. *Message of the President, Aug. 29, 1862.* [Richmond, 1862]. Boston Athenaeum. http://catalog.bostonathenaeum.org/vwebv/holdingsInfo ?bibId=481258. Accessed Jan. 20, 2019.

———. *The Rise and Fall of the Confederate Government.* 2 vols. New York: D. Appleton, 1881.

Davis, William C. "General Samuel Cooper." In *Leaders of the Lost Cause: New Perspectives on the Confederate High Command*, edited by Gary W. Gallagher and Joseph T. Glatthaar, 101–32. Mechanicsburg, PA: Stackpole, 2004.

DeLeon, Perry M. "Military Record of the DeLeon Family and of Captain Perry M. DeLeon." *Publications of the American Jewish Historical Society* 50, no. 4 (June 1961): 332–34.

DeLeon, Thomas C. *Four Years in Rebel Capitals.* Mobile, AL: Gossip Printing, 1892.

"Description of the Model for the Proposed Monument to Be Erected to Surgeon-General Samuel Preston Moore, Confederate States Army." *Southern Practitioner* 33, no. 4 (Apr. 1911): 203–12.

"Discussion on Opium." In *Proceedings of the American Pharmaceutical Association at the Thirteenth Annual Meeting Held in Boston, Mass., September, 1865*, 51–52. Philadelphia: Merrihew & Son, 1865.

Dorris, Jonathan Truman. *Pardon and Amnesty: The Restoration of the Confederates to Their Rights and Privileges, 1861–1898.* Chapel Hill: University of North Carolina Press, 1953.

"Dr. James B. McCaw." In *Transactions of the Thirty-Seventh Annual Session of the Medical Society of Virginia*, 305–6. Richmond: Williams Printing, 1906.

"Dudley Dunn Saunders, M.D." *Journal of the Tennessee State Medical Association* 1, no. 8 (Jan. 1909): 311–13.

Edmonson, James M. *American Surgical Instruments: An Illustrated History of Their Manufacture and a Directory of Instrument Makers to 1900*. San Francisco: Norman, 1997.

Elzas, Barnett A. *The Jews of South Carolina*. Philadelphia: J. B. Lippincott, 1905.

England, Joseph W. "The American Manufacture of Quinine Sulphate." *Alumni Report* (Philadelphia College of Pharmacy) 34 (Mar. 1898): 57–64.

Epstein, Robert M. "The Creation and Evolution of the Army Corps in the American Civil War." *Journal of Military History* 55, no. 1 (Jan. 1991): 21–46.

Estill, Mary S., ed. "Diary of a Confederate Congressman, 1862–1863." Pt. 1. *Southwestern Historical Quarterly* 38, no. 4 (Apr. 1935): 270–301.

Farr, Warner Dahlgren. "Samuel Preston Moore: Confederate Surgeon General." *Civil War History* 41, no. 1 (Mar. 1995): 41–56.

Faust, Drew Gilpin. *This Republic of Suffering: Death and the American Civil War*. New York: Vintage, 2008.

Felt, Jeremy P. "Lucius B. Northrop and the Confederacy's Subsistence Department." *Virginia Magazine of History and Biography* 69, no. 2 (Apr. 1961): 181–93.

Freedley, Edwin T., ed. *Leading Pursuits and Leading Men: A Treatise on the Principle Trades and Manufactures of the United States*. Philadelphia: Edward Young, 1854.

Freeman, Douglas Southall. *A Calendar of Confederate Papers*. Richmond: Confederate Museum, 1908.

"The French Field-Hospitals, or Ambulances." *London Lancet* 1, no. 4 (Apr. 1855): 374–76.

Futch, Ovid L. *History of Andersonville Prison*. Gainesville: University of Florida Press, 1968.

Gaillard, Edwin S. "In Memoriam." *Richmond and Louisville Medical Journal* 23, no. 4 (Apr. 1877): 401–2.

———. "The Medical and Surgical Lessons of the Late War." *New Eclectic Magazine* 4 (June 1869): 705–18.

Gaston, J. McFadden. "Personal and Surgical Reminiscences of the War." *Atlanta Medical and Surgical Journal* 13, no. 3 (May 1896): 161–71.

General Directions for Collecting and Drying Medicinal Substances of the Vegetable Kingdom. Richmond: Surgeon General's Office, 1862.

The General Military Hospital for the North Carolina Troops in Petersburg Virginia. Raleigh: Strother & Marcom, 1861.

George Scarborough Barnsley Papers. In *Records of Ante-Bellum Southern Plantations from the Revolution through the Civil War,* edited by Kenneth M. Stampp. Ser. J, *Selections from the Southern Historical Collection, Manuscripts Department, Library of the University of North Carolina at Chapel Hill.* Pt. 4, *Georgia and Florida.* Bethesda, MD: University Publications of America, 1989. Microfilm, roll 43.

Georgia Relief and Hospital Association. *Report of the Executive Committee, October 29, 1862.* Augusta, GA: Steam Press of Chronicle & Sentinel, 1862.

Gholson, S. C. "Recollections of My First Six Months in the Confederate Army." *Southern Practitioner* 27, no. 1 (Jan. 1905): 32–43.

Gildersleeve, John R. "History of Chimborazo Hospital, Richmond, Va., and its Medical Officers during 1861–1865." *Virginia Medical Semi-Monthly* 9, no. 7 (July 8, 1904): 148–54.

Gillett, Mary C. *The Army Medical Department, 1818–1865.* Washington, DC: US Army Center of Military History, 1987.

Griffith, Lucille. "Mrs. Juliet Opie Hopkins and Alabama Military Hospitals." *Alabama Review* 6, no. 2 (Apr. 1953): 99–120.

Gross, Samuel D. *A Manual of Military Surgery; or, Hints on the Emergencies of Field, Camp and Hospital Practice.* Philadelphia: Lippincott, 1861; Augusta, GA: Chronicle & Sentinel, 1861; Richmond: J. W. Randolph, 1862.

———. "A Manual of Military Surgery; or, Hints on the Emergencies of Field, Camp, and Hospital Practice." *Southern Medical and Surgical Journal* 17, no. 7 (July 1861): 529–85; no. 8 (Aug. 1861): 619–40.

Hambrecht, F. Terry. "J. J. Chisolm, M.D.: Confederate Medical and Surgical Innovator." In Schmidt and Hasegawa, *Years of Change and Suffering,* 69–87.

Hasegawa, Guy R. "'Absurd Prejudice': A. Snowden Piggot and the Confederate Medical Laboratory at Lincolnton." *North Carolina Historical Review* 81, no. 3 (July 2004): 313–34.

———. *Mending Broken Soldiers: The Union and Confederate Programs to Supply Artificial Limbs.* Carbondale: Southern Illinois University Press, 2012.

———. "Quinine Substitutes in the Confederate Army." *Military Medicine* 172, no. 6 (June 2007): 650–55.

———. "Southern Resources, Southern Medicines." In Schmidt and Hasegawa, *Years of Change and Suffering,* 107–25.

Hasegawa, Guy R., and F. Terry Hambrecht. "The Confederate Medical Laboratories." *Southern Medical Journal* 96, no. 12 (Dec. 2003): 1221–30.

Hesseltine, William B. *Civil War Prisons: A Study in War Psychology.* Columbus: Ohio State University Press, 1930. Reprint, New York: Frederick Ungar, 1964.

Hicks, Robert D. "Scabrous Matters: Spurious Vaccination in the Confederate Army." In *War Matters: Material Culture in the Civil War Era*, edited by Joan E. Cashin, 123–50. Chapel Hill: University of North Carolina Press, 2018.

Hilde, Libra R. *Worth a Dozen Men: Women and Nursing in the Civil War South.* Charlottesville: University of Virginia Press, 2012.

Holloway, James M. "Reminiscences of a Surgeon in the Confederate States Service." *Lost Cause* 3, no. 1 (Aug. 1899): 1–3.

Huse, Caleb. *The Supplies for the Confederate Army: How They Were Obtained in Europe and How Paid For.* Boston: T. R. Marvin & Son, 1904.

"In Memoriam." *Richmond and Louisville Medical Journal* 25, no. 1 (Jan. 1878): 101–2.

Johnson, Ludwell H. "Beverly Tucker's Canadian Mission, 1864–1865." *Journal of Southern History* 29, no. 1 (Feb. 1963): 88–99.

———. "Trading with the Union: The Evolution of Confederate Policy." *Virginia Magazine of History and Biography* 78, no. 3 (July 1970): 308–25.

Johnson, Rossiter, ed. *The Twentieth Century Biographical Dictionary of Notable Americans.* Vol. 3, *Cowan–Erich.* Boston: Biographical Society, 1904.

Jones, John B. *A Rebel War Clerk's Diary.* Edited by James I. Robertson Jr. 2 vols. Lawrence: University Press of Kansas, 2015.

Jones, Joseph. "Investigations upon the Diseases of the Federal Prisoners Confined in Camp Sumter, Andersonville, Ga." In *Sanitary Memoirs of the War of the Rebellion*, 469–655. New York: US Sanitary Commission, 1867.

———. "Investigations upon the Nature, Causes, and Treatment of Hospital Gangrene, as It Prevailed in the Confederate Armies, 1861–1865." In *Surgical Memoirs of the War of the Rebellion*, 143–570. New York: US Sanitary Commission, 1871.

———. "Medical Corps of the Confederate Army and Navy, 1861–1865." *Atlanta Medical and Surgical Journal* 7, no. 6 (Aug. 1890): 339–53.

Journal of the Congress of the Confederate States of America, 1861–1865. 7 vols. 58th Cong., 2nd sess., 1904–5, S. Doc. 234.

Koonce, Donald B., ed. *Doctor to the Front: The Recollections of Confederate Surgeon Thomas Fanning Wood, 1861–1865.* Knoxville: University of Tennessee Press, 2000.

Koste, Jodi L. "'Medical School for a Nation': The Medical College of Virginia, 1860–1865." In Schmidt and Hasegawa, *Years of Change and Suffering*, 13–35.

Krick, Robert E. L. *Staff Officers in Gray: A Biographical Register of the Staff Officers in the Army of Northern Virginia.* Chapel Hill: University of North Carolina Press, 2003.

Lane, Alexander G. "The Winder Hospital, of Richmond, Va." *Southern Practitioner* 26, no. 1 (Jan. 1904): 35–41.

Larrey, Dominique Jean. *Memoirs of Military Surgery.* Translated by Richard Willmott Hall. Vol. 1. Baltimore: Joseph Cushing, 1814.

Leigh, Philip. *Trading with the Enemy: The Covert Economy during the American Civil War.* Yardley, PA: Westholme, 2014.

Letterman, Jonathan. *Medical Recollections of the Army of the Potomac.* New York: D. Appleton, 1866.

Lewis, Samuel E. "Samuel Preston Moore, M.D., Surgeon General of the Confederate States." *Southern Practitioner* 23, no. 8 (Aug. 1901): 381–86.

Longmore, Sir Thomas. *A Treatise on the Transport of Sick and Wounded Troops.* London: Her Majesty's Stationery Office, 1869.

Mackall, W. W. "The Late Doctor Francis Sorrel." *Georgia Historical Quarterly* 1, no. 1 (Mar. 1917): 36–39.

Macleod, George H. B. *Notes on the Surgery of the War in the Crimea.* London: John Churchill, 1858; Richmond: J. W. Randolph, 1862.

Mallory, Stephen R. "Last Days of the Confederate Government." *McClure's Magazine* 16, no. 2 (Dec. 1900): 99–107; no. 3 (Jan. 1901): 239–48.

A Manual of Military Surgery, Prepared for the Use of the Confederate States Army. Richmond: Ayres & Wade, 1863.

Maury, R. B. "Hypodermic Injections in the Treatment of Disease." *American Journal of Medical Sciences,* n.s., 52, no. 104 (Oct. 1866): 371–73.

The Medical and Surgical History of the War of the Rebellion. 3 vols. in 6 pts. Washington, DC: Government Printing Office, 1870–88.

"The Medical Department of the Confederate States Army—Its Relation to the Other Branches of the Service, and the Duties of its Officers." *Confederate States Medical and Surgical Journal* 1, no. 2 (Feb. 1864): 26.

Mitchell, John K. *Charge to the Graduates of Jefferson Medical College of Philadelphia; Delivered March 7, 1857.* Philadelphia: T. K. and P. G. Collins, 1857.

Monteiro, Aristides. *War Reminiscences by the Surgeon of Mosby's Command.* Richmond: Everett Waddey, 1890.

Moore, Samuel Preston. "Address of the President of the Association of Medical Officers of Confederate States Army and Navy." *Southern Practitioner* 31, no. 10 (Oct. 1909): 491–98.

Munson, E. B., ed. *Confederate Incognito: The Civil War Reports of "Long Grabs,"* a.k.a. Murdoch John McSween, 26th and 35th North Carolina Infantry. Jefferson, NC: McFarland, 2013.

"Necrology: Herman Baer." *South Carolina Historical and Genealogical Magazine* 2, no. 2 (Apr. 1901): 166.

"Necrology: James T. Meek, M.D." *Journal of the American Medical Association* 7, no. 25 (Dec. 18, 1886): 697.

The New American Cyclopedia: A Popular Dictionary of General Knowledge. Edited by George Ripley and Charles A. Dana. 8 vols. New York: D. Appleton, 1859.

Newton, Edwin D. "My Recollections and Reminiscences." *Southern Practitioner* 30, no. 8 (Oct. 1908): 474–89.

Nichols, F. B. "Review of the New York Markets, from March 24th to April 24th, 1861." *American Druggists' Circular and Chemical Gazette* 5 (May 1861): 112.

Nightingale, Florence. *Notes on Hospitals.* London: John W. Parker & Son, 1859.

Norris, David A. "'For the Benefit of Our Gallant Volunteers': North Carolina's State Medical Department and Civilian Volunteer Efforts, 1861–1862." *North Carolina Historical Review* 75, no. 3 (July 1998): 297–326.

"Obituary Record: Dr. Samuel Preston Moore." *Virginia Medical Monthly* 16, no. 3 (June 1889): 250–54.

"Obituary Record: Dr. William Middleton Michel." *Virginia Medical Monthly* 21, no. 4 (July 1894): 379–80.

Official Army Register, for 1856. Washington, DC: Adjutant General's Office, 1856.

Official Army Register, for 1861. Washington, DC: Adjutant General's Office, 1861.

Official Army Register, for 1862. Washington, DC: Adjutant General's Office, 1862.

Parker, William Harwar. *Recollections of a Naval Officer, 1841–1865.* New York: Charles Scribners' Sons, 1883. Reprinted, with introduction and notes by Craig L. Symonds, Annapolis, MD: Naval Institute Press, 1985.

Parrish, Edward, and William C. Bakes. "Notes on Lactucarium and Its Preparations." *American Journal of Pharmacy* 32 (May 1860): 225–30.

Payne, John W. "Samuel Preston Moore's Letters to William E. Woodruff." *Arkansas Historical Quarterly* 15, no. 3 (Autumn 1956): 228–48.

Pember, Phoebe Yates. *A Southern Woman's Story.* New York: G. W Carleton, 1879.

Porcher, Francis Peyre. "Confederate Surgeons." *Southern Historical Society Papers* 17 (1889): 12–21.

———. *Resources of the Southern Fields and Forests, Medical, Economical, and Agricultural.* Charleston, SC: Evans & Cogswell, 1863; Richmond: West & Johnston, 1863.

"Proceedings of the Association of Medical Officers of the Army and Navy of the Confederacy—Fourteenth Annual Session." *Southern Practitioner* 33, no. 8 (Aug. 1911): 410–18.

"The Prospect before Us." *Confederate States Medical and Surgical Journal* 1, no. 5 (May 1864): 78.

Ramsdell, Charles W., ed. *Laws and Joint Resolutions of the Last Session of the Confederate Congress*. Durham, NC: Duke University Press, 1941.

Report of the Secretary of the Treasury, Transmitting a Report of the Commerce and Navigation of the United States, for the Year Ending June 30, 1859. Washington, DC: William A. Harris, 1859.

"Revival of Medical Journalism." *American Medical Times*, n.s., 9, no. 1 (July 2, 1864): 9.

Richardson, James D. *A Compilation of the Messages and Papers of the Confederacy*. Vol. 1. Nashville: United States Publishing, 1906.

Roberts, Deering J. "Confederate Medical Service." In Thompson, *Prisons and Hospitals*, 238–50.

———. "Organization and Personnel of the Medical Department of the Confederacy." In Thompson, *Prisons and Hospitals*, 349–52.

Rosenberg, Charles E. *The Care of Strangers: The Rise of America's Hospital System*. New York: Basic Books, 1987.

Rothstein, William G. *American Medical Schools and the Practice of Medicine: A History*. New York: Oxford University Press, 1987.

Rowland, Dunbar, ed. *Jefferson Davis, Constitutionalist: His Letters, Papers, and Speeches*. Vol. 8. Jackson: Mississippi Department of Archives and History, 1923.

"Salutatory." *Confederate States Medical and Surgical Journal* 1, no. 1 (Jan. 1864): 13.

Sanders, Charles W., Jr. *While in the Hands of the Enemy*. Baton Rouge: Louisiana State University Press, 2005.

Schmidt, James M., and Guy R. Hasegawa, eds. *Years of Change and Suffering: Modern Perspectives on Civil War Medicine*. Roseville, MN: Edinborough, 2009.

Schroeder-Lein, Glenna R. *Confederate Hospitals on the Move: Samuel H. Stout and the Army of Tennessee*. Columbia: University of South Carolina Press, 1994.

Sheriff & Chataigne's Richmond City Directory. Richmond: West, Johnston, 1874.

Sheriff & Co.'s Richmond City Directory. Richmond: West, Johnston, 1876.

Slawson, Robert G. "Medical Training in the United States Prior to the Civil War." *Journal of Evidence-Based Complementary and Alternative Medicine* 17, no. 1 (Jan. 1, 2012): 11–27.

Smart, Charles. "Transportation of Wounded in War." In *Proceedings of the Fourth Annual Meeting of the Association of Military Surgeons of the United States*. St. Louis: Buxton & Skinner, 1894.

"The Soldier-Surgeon." *Dublin University Magazine* 45, no. 267 (Mar. 1855): 253–77.

Soley, James Russell. *The Blockade and the Cruisers*. New York: Charles Scribner's Sons, 1883.

Sorrel, Francis. "Gun-Shot Wounds—Army of Northern Virginia." *Confederate States Medical and Surgical Journal* 1, no. 10 (Oct. 1864): 153–55.

Sorrel, G. Moxley. *Recollections of a Confederate Staff Officer*. New York: Neale, 1905.

Squibb, Edward R. "The Drug Inspectors and the Profession." *American Medical Times* 2 (Jan. 26, 1861): 66–68.

Standard Supply Table of the Indigenous Remedies for Field Service, and the Sick in General Hospitals. Richmond, 1863.

Stout, Samuel H. "Dental Surgeons in the Armies and Navies." *Texas Medical Journal* 15, no. 3 (Sept. 1899): 132–34.

———. "On the Best Models and Most Easily Constructed Military Hospital Wards for Temporary Use in War." In *Transactions of the International Medical Congress*, edited by John B. Hamilton, 2:88–91. Washington, DC: Wm. F. Fell, 1887.

———. "Some Facts of the History of the Organization of the Medical Service of the Confederate Armies and Hospitals." Pts. 10, 13, 16–19, 22, 23. *Southern Practitioner* 24, no. 3 (Mar. 1902): 159–64; no. 11 (Nov. 1902): 622–26; 25, no. 2 (Feb. 1903): 91–98; no. 3 (Mar. 1903); 155–61; no. 4 (Apr. 1903): 215–22; no. 5 (May 1903): 274–83; no. 9 (Sept. 1903): 517–26; no. 10 (Oct. 1903): 566–74.

The Stranger's Guide and Official Directory for the City of Richmond. Richmond: Geo. P. Evans, 1863.

Thompson, Holland, ed. *Prisons and Hospitals*. Vol. 7 of *The Photographic History of the Civil War*, edited by Francis Trevelyan Miller. New York: Review of Reviews, 1911.

Thompson, Holland. "Treatment of Prisoners." In Thompson, *Prisons and Hospitals*, 156–86. New York: Review of Reviews, 1911.

Thompson, Samuel Bernard. *Confederate Purchasing Operations Abroad*. Gloucester, MA: Peter Smith, 1973.

"To the Reader." *Confederate States Medical and Surgical Journal* 1, no. 9 (Sept. 1864): 140.

Tower, R. Lockwood, ed. *Lee's Adjutant: The Wartime Letters of Colonel Walter Herron Taylor, 1862–1865*. Columbia: University of South Carolina Press, 1995.

Trial of Henry Wirz. 40th Cong., 2nd sess., 1868. H. Exec. Doc. 23.

Tucker, Jane Ellis. *Beverly Tucker: A Memoir by His Wife*. Richmond: Frank Baptist, [1893?].

Van Buren, William H., and C. R. Agnew. "Report No. 23, July 31, 1861." In *Documents of the U.S. Sanitary Commission*, vol. 1. New York: US Sanitary Commission, 1866.

Vandiver, Frank E., ed. *Confederate Blockade Running through Bermuda, 1861–1865: Letters and Cargo Manifests*. Austin: University of Texas Press, 1947.

———. *Ploughshares into Swords: Josiah Gorgas and Confederate Ordnance*. College Station: Texas A&M University Press, 1994.

———. *Rebel Brass: The Confederate Command System*. Baton Rouge: Louisiana State University Press, 1956.

Vanfelson, Charles A. *The Little Red Book or Department Directory*. Richmond: Tyler, Wise, & Allegre, 1861.

Van Riper, Paul P., and Harry N. Scheiber. "The Confederate Civil Service." *Journal of Southern History* 25, no. 4 (Nov. 1959): 448–70.

Wailes, L. A. "A Case of Field Surgery." *Confederate Veteran* 25, no. 3 (Mar. 1917): 107.

War Department (Confederate). *Army Regulations, Adopted for the Use of the Army of the Confederate States, in Accordance with Late Acts of Congress*. Richmond: West & Johnston, 1861.

———. *Regulations for the Army of the Confederate States, 1862* (Mar. 13, 1862). Richmond: J. W. Randolph, 1862.

———. *Regulations for the Army of the Confederate States, 1862* (Nov. 1, 1862). Richmond: West & Johnston, 1862.

———. *Regulations for the Army of the Confederate States, 1863* (Jan. 28, 1863). Richmond: J. W. Randolph, 1863.

———. *Regulations for the Army of the Confederate States, 1864*. 3rd ed. Richmond: J. W. Randolph, 1864.

———. *Regulations for the Army of the Confederate States, as Adopted by Act of Congress, Approved March 6, 1861*. New Orleans: Henry P. Lathrop, 1861.

———. *Regulations for the Medical Department of the Confederate States Army*. Richmond: Ritchie & Dunnavant, 1861.

———. *Regulations for the Medical Department of the C.S. Army* (Apr. 10, 1862). Richmond: Ritchie & Dunnavant, 1862.

———. *Regulations for the Medical Department of the C.S. Army* (Mar. 25, 1863). Richmond: Ritchie & Dunnavant, 1863.

War Department (US). *Regulations for the Army of the United States, 1857*. New York: Harper & Brothers, 1857.

———. *Regulations for the Medical Department of the Army*. Washington, DC: George W. Bowman, 1860.

Warner, John Harley. *The Therapeutic Perspective: Medical Practice, Knowledge, and Identity in America, 1820–1885*. Princeton, NJ: Princeton University Press, 1997.

The War of the Rebellion: A Compilation of the Official Records of the Union and Confederate Armies. 70 vols. in 128 pts. Washington, DC: Government Printing Office, 1880–1901.

Warren, Edward. *A Doctor's Experiences in Three Continents*. Baltimore: Cushings & Bailey, 1885.

———. *An Epitome of Practical Surgery, for Field and Hospital*. Richmond: West & Johnston, 1863.

Watson, Irving A., ed. *Physicians and Surgeons of America*. Concord, NH: Republican Press Association, 1896.

Welsh, Jack D. *Two Confederate Hospitals and Their Patients: Atlanta to Opelika*. Macon, GA: Mercer University Press, 2005.

Wiernik, Peter. *History of the Jews in America*. New York: Jewish Press Publishing, 1912.

Williams, Edward B., ed. *Rebel Brothers: The Civil War Letters of the Truehearts*. College Station: Texas A&M University Press, 1995.

Williams, Mrs. James H. "Reminiscences of a Clerk in the Medical Purveyor's Office and in the Treasury of the Confederate Government Richmond, Virginia." *Southern Practitioner* 39, no. 7 (July 1917): 301–5.

Wilson, Harold S. *Confederate Industry: Manufacturers and Quartermasters in the Civil War*. Jackson: University Press of Mississippi, 2002.

Wise, Stephen R. *Lifeline of the Confederacy: Blockade Running during the Civil War*. Columbia: University of South Carolina Press, 1988.

Wood, C. A., and Co. "Review of the Drug Trade of New York for 1859." In *Annual Report of the Chamber of Commerce of the State of New-York, for the Year 1859–'60*, 212–16. New York: John W. Amerman, 1860.

Wood, C. A., and F. B. Nichols. "Annual Report on Drugs for the Year 1860." In *Third Annual Report of the Chamber of Commerce of the State of New York, for the Year 1860–'61*, 303–9. New York: John W. Amerman, 1861.

———. "Review of the Drug Trade of New York." In *Fourth Annual Report of the Chamber of Commerce of the State of New York, for the Year 1861–'62*, 164–72. New York: John W. Amerman, 1862.

Wood, Thomas F. "Otis Frederick Manson, M.D." *North Carolina Medical Journal* 21, no. 3 (Mar. 1888): 150–62.

———. "Surgeon General S. P. Moore." *North Carolina Medical Journal* 23, no. 5 (May 1889): 400.

Woodward, C. Vann, and Elisabeth Muhlenfeld, eds. *The Private Mary Chesnut: The Unpublished Civil War Diaries*. New York: Oxford University Press, 1984.

Wright, Daniel F. "The Effects of the Hunterian Method of Ligation on Inflammation." *Confederate States Medical and Surgical Journal* 1, no. 11 (Nov. 1864): 177–78.

Year Book, 1909–1910 of the Confederate Memorial Literary Society. Richmond: Whittet & Shepperson, 1910.

Year Book, 1911–1912 of the Confederate Memorial Literary Society. Richmond: Whittet & Shepperson, 1912.

Yearns, Wilfred Buck. *The Confederate Congress*. Athens: University of Georgia Press, 1960.

Zeilin, J. H. "Drug Business in the Late Confederate States." In *Proceedings of the National Wholesale Druggists Association, in Conventional at Indianapolis, Oct. 22, 23, 24, 25, 1889*, 182–86. Minneapolis: Swinburne, 1890.

Index

Page numbers in italics indicate illustrations.

Guy R. Hasegawa, a retired pharmacist and editor, is the author of *Villainous Compounds: Chemical Weapons and the American Civil War* and *Mending Broken Soldiers: The Union and Confederate Programs to Supply Artificial Limbs.* He has written numerous book chapters and articles on Civil War medicine and has served on the board of directors of the National Museum of Civil War Medicine and the Society of Civil War Surgeons.

ENGAGING
—*the*—
CIVIL WAR

Engaging the Civil War, a series founded by the historians at the blog Emerging Civil War (www.emergingcivilwar.com), adopts the sensibility and accessibility of public history while adhering to the standards of academic scholarship. To engage readers and bring them to a new understanding of America's great story, series authors draw on insights they gained while working with the public—walking the ground where history happened at battlefields and historic sites, talking with visitors in museums, and educating students in classrooms. With fresh perspectives, field-tested ideas, and in-depth research, volumes in the series connect readers with the story of the Civil War in ways that make history meaningful to them while underscoring the continued relevance of the war, its causes, and its effects. All Americans can claim the Civil War as part of their history. This series , which was cofounded by Chris Mackowski and Kristopher D. White, helps them engage with it.

Chris Mackowski and Brian Matthew Jordan, Series Editors

Queries and submissions
emergingcivilwar@gmail.com